A Guide to Asperger Syndrome

Asperger syndrome is an autism spectrum disorder, usually with life-long consequences for social interaction and behaviour. The disorder is neurodevelopmental and symptoms appear in the preschool years. Individuals affected are often misunderstood and sometimes misdiagnosed when they apply for help.

A Guide to Asperger Syndrome is an accessible handbook for all those touched by Asperger syndrome, one of the most common variants of disorders in the so-called autism spectrum. In it, Christopher Gillberg, a world-renowned authority in the field, gives an in-depth account of symptoms, diagnosis, prevalence, background factors, prognosis and intervention. The book is intended for a wide readership, including those affected, their families, and clinicians working with children, adolescents and adults with psychological, developmental, behavioural or psychiatric problems.

Christopher Gillberg is Professor of Child and Adolescent Psychiatry at the University of Göteborg in Sweden, and St George's Hospital Medical School, London, UK.

A Guide to
Asperger Syndrome

Christopher Gillberg

University of Göteborg, Sweden, and
St George's Hospital Medical School, London, UK

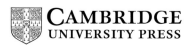

CAMBRIDGE
UNIVERSITY PRESS

PUBLISHED BY THE PRESS SYNDICATE OF THE UNIVERSITY OF CAMBRIDGE
The Pitt Building, Trumpington Street, Cambridge, United Kingdom

CAMBRIDGE UNIVERSITY PRESS
The Edinburgh Building, Cambridge CB2 2RU, UK
40 West 20th Street, New York, NY 10011-4211, USA
477 Williamstown Road, Port Melbourne, VIC 3207, Australia
Ruiz de Alarcón 13, 28014 Madrid, Spain
Dock House, The Waterfront, Cape Town 8001, South Africa

http://www.cambridge.org

Printed in the United Kingdom at the University Press, Cambridge

Typeface Minion 11/14.5pt   *System* Poltype® [v n]

A catalogue record for this book is available from the British Library

Library of Congress Cataloguing in Publication Data available

ISBN 0 521 00183 8 paperback

Every effort has been made in preparing this book to provide accurate and up-to-date information which is in
accord with accepted standards and practice at the time of publication. Nevertheless, the authors, editors and
publisher can make no warranties that the information contained herein is totally free from error, not least
because clinical standards are constantly changing through research and regulation. The authors, editors and
publisher therefore disclaim all liability for direct or consequential damages resulting from the use of material
contained in this book. Readers are strongly advised to pay careful attention to information provided by the
manufacturer of any drugs or equipment that they plan to use.

Contents

Preface

This book is intended for all those who struggle with Asperger syndrome in their everyday life. They are many. They range from the people with the diagnosis, and their near and dear, through clinicians faced with the problems of understanding, investigating and intervening in 'a disorder' that they heard little about during their education, but read about in the newspapers and magazines almost on a weekly basis.

Asperger syndrome achieved its status as a specific diagnostic entity about 20 years ago. It was only after the death of the Austrian paediatrician Hans Asperger, that 'his' syndrome received widespread recognition outside central Europe. In 1981, Lorna Wing, a British autism expert, published a paper in which she coined the term 'Asperger's syndrome'. Asperger himself had referred to the condition as 'autistic psychopathy', which would probably best translate as 'autistic personality disorder' in present-day terminology. His first paper on the syndrome appeared in 1944, only months after Leo Kanner published his first report on 'early infantile autism'. Almost 20 years before Asperger, the Russian scientific assistant in neurology Ewa Ssucharewa, wrote a paper in which she referred to 'schizoid psychopathy' (personality disorder) in children. It seems clear that she was describing the same condition that Asperger called 'autistic personality disorder'. Nevertheless, it is Asperger's name that is now attached to the constellation of symptoms/personality traits that are at the core of the present volume.

Asperger syndrome is usually congenital or, rarely, contracted after brain injury in the first few years of life. It is a 'neuropsychiatric' syndrome – or, perhaps, rather a constellation of traits of unusual development of the nervous system, a 'variation' of brain development – in the sense that there are psychological, behavioural, emotional and cognitive characteristics that have a biological basis. Symptoms (or 'features') of the condition, albeit sometimes subtle, are present from early childhood, but it is still common for people affected to seek psychiatric or other medical help only in adult age. In fact, many with the 'classic Asperger personality' never seek help specifically for their 'Asperger problems'.

Asperger syndrome is already known among portions of the lay community. Some parents apply for psychiatric help for their child with the specific concern: does my child have Asperger syndrome? Many clinicians know little more, indeed sometimes less, than these parents about the condition, and it is not uncommon for misunderstandings to occur in this context. Only a small number of books have so far been published specifically on Asperger syndrome, and the few that have appeared are mostly directed either at clinicians *or* parents or have been written by people affected by the condition, providing highly personal accounts. This volume is intended for a larger readership. I hope that it will be useful for *all* those concerned. A common knowledge base is the best investment when it comes to dealing with problems and strengths in neuropsychiatric conditions/disorders and syndromes of unusual development. This book aims to stimulate the development of such a common, indeed general, knowledge base about Asperger syndrome in the community at large.

Throughout the text I shall be referring to 'people' ('individuals', 'children', 'teenagers', 'adults') *with* Asperger syndrome, not 'Asperger people'. I know that there are those who find a rigorous avoidance of the latter term amusing or even ridiculous. However, I believe that by separating the syndrome/condition from the people who have it, one can, to some extent, keep track of what it is in a person's behaviour and experience that is attributable to the 'syndrome', and what it is that is linked rather to *being an individual member of humankind.* It is, unfortunately, much too common that individuals with a condition such as Asperger syndrome are all 'treated as one', that beliefs are held about 'such people', and that the enormous variability, indeed the uniqueness of each person with the condition is overlooked. However, this is not to say that the *syndrome* is not characteristic or that it is less 'real' than other medical conditions or symptom constellations.

This book is dedicated to all the hundreds of individuals with Asperger syndrome whom I have met throughout the years, patients, people of genius, 'nerds', loners, comedians, artists, writers and scientists, people on the borders of 'normality' (whatever that is). They have taught me more about human development – including normal development – than any psychiatry or psychology textbook. They are, in spite of their difficulties, an enormous asset to humankind, and so this volume is not just about the drawbacks, but also about the strengths and the positive aspects of Asperger syndrome.

Christopher Gillberg

Göteborg

1

Introduction

Hans Asperger appears to have been unaware of the writings of Ewa Ssucharewa when he published his first paper on the condition that he referred to as 'autistic psychopathy' in 1944. Indeed, there is no indication that he ever learnt about the 1926 publication by the Russian neurology scientific assistant about a condition that she referred to as 'schizoid personality of childhood'. Reading Asperger's case histories on boys with 'autistic personality disorder' (which is really what is meant by 'autistic psychopathy') and Ssucharewa's on boys with 'schizoid personality disorder', one is struck by the great similarity rather than by any major difference. It seems clear that the two physicians were really describing the same phenomenon. However, Ssucharewa's publication was not brought to the attention of the international research community until 1995 (by Sula Wolff, a Scottish psychiatrist). Asperger's report had been widely cited long before that – and most notably by Lorna Wing, the British autism expert – and so his name has become attached to the syndrome.

It is of historical interest that Leo Kanner, the US psychiatrist who first reported on the 'classic' variant of childhood autism as a syndrome in 1943, never once mentioned Asperger, but did refer, albeit in passing (in 1971) to Ssucharewa. Asperger, on the other hand, referred to Kanner, but felt that 'autistic psychopathy' was clearly different from the syndrome that Kanner had described.

The first annotated translation into English of Asperger's original paper was published in 1991, and it is only in the past 10 years that Asperger syndrome has become widely discussed in child and adolescent psychiatry and by the public in general. A few years ago, interest in the condition sparked also in developmental paediatrics ('neuropaediatrics', 'child neurology') and in adult (including forensic) psychiatry.

Hans Asperger worked as a paediatrician in Vienna and gradually became absorbed by deviant/unusual development in children. He was also an ardent proponent of so-called *Heilpädagogik*. In his clinic, educational modes of intervention dominated, particularly as regards young boys with social interaction difficulties and behaviour problems. Asperger lectured about 'his boys' in the 1930s, but published his first paper on the condition (in German) only in 1944. Possibly because of its roots in the German culture and language during the second world war, Asperger's paper was not widely discussed outside of central Europe – even though 'autistic psychopathy' was part at least of Scandinavian and Dutch child psychiatry nomenclature from the 1970s onwards. It was also referred to in the major British child psychiatry textbook edited by Rutter and Hersov in 1977.

Leo Kanner, on the other hand, wrote in English and worked in the United States, and his work on 'autistic disturbances of affective contact', soon termed 'early infantile autism', became widely known across the world. His first paper (1943) on 11 children (8 boys and 3 girls) described a condition, with very early – even infantile – onset, characterised by extreme difficulties in reciprocal social interaction and a pattern of elaborate repetitive routines or 'insistence on sameness'. Looking back, it has become clear that Kanner and Asperger were referring to very similar conditions. However, Kanner's cases were usually of low intelligence (although occasionally with some islets of extraordinary ability), whereas Asperger's patients – at least in the vast majority of cases – had normal or very high intelligence levels.

It has been said about Asperger that he had a special affinity for children with autistic psychopathy because he himself had many – perhaps all – the personality features considered typical of the condition. It is not clear that this was the case, but, according to his daughter, who I interviewed together with Uta Frith, a British autism expert, in 1990, there were several examples of exaggerated formalism, a 'stiff' attitude in social relationships and a need for routines bordering on the extreme.

A Dutch physician, Arn van Krevelen, in the late 1960s and early 1970s tried to draw attention to Asperger's writings by comparing autistic psychopathy with Kanner's variant of autism. However, it was not until a year after Asperger's death, when Lorna Wing (1981) published her account of 34 cases of what she referred to as 'Asperger's syndrome', that interest in his work started to grow globally. In the United States, the condition was not recognised as a specific diagnostic entity until the publication of the fourth edition of the *Diagnostic and Statistical Manual of Mental Disorders* (DSM-IV) in 1994 (where it is referred to as Asperger's disorder).

Over the past decade, hundreds of scientific papers have been published on Asperger syndrome/Asperger's disorder. During the same period, knowledge has grown immensely with regard to brain functioning and brain dysfunction. It has even become possible to study the brain mechanisms that may underlie Asperger syndrome. Developments in neighbouring fields have also contributed both to a better understanding of Asperger syndrome, and also to a more complex and complicated picture altogether. Results from studies on high-functioning autism, semantic-pragmatic disorders, non-verbal learning disability, right-hemisphere dysfunction, pathological demand avoidance, obsessive-compulsive personality disorder, tics and Tourette syndrome, deficits in attention, motor control and perception (DAMP), attention-deficit/hyperactivity disorder (ADHD), and on girls with social deficits and learning problems, have all combined to produce the concept of a rather broad 'autism spectrum'. Many of these terms are relatively new and refer to conditions/disabilities that lead to symptoms and handicap that overlap and share many features with those of Asperger syndrome.

These days, Asperger syndrome is one of the most widely discussed diagnoses in psychiatry, not just in child psychiatry, but in adult services also. It is clear that many adult psychiatric patients presenting major diagnostic difficulty actually have – previously undiagnosed – Asperger syndrome. Asperger syndrome is no longer a very rare diagnosis in child psychiatry. Teachers come across cases in their everyday practice, not just once in a blue moon, but on a rather regular basis. People with all the hallmarks of Asperger syndrome who were never diagnosed read about the symptoms and typical features in some article and realise that they correspond to their own problems and assets. Parents understand, sometimes without consulting any expert in the field, that their children may be suffering from Asperger syndrome. Spouses realise that their partner 'has Asperger's'.

In this kind of setting, it is important that the information available is factual and easy to access. This is the context in which this book has been written. I have worked with patients and questions relating to the field of high-functioning autism and Asperger syndrome for more than 25 years. My first patient with the condition was a proband in a research project about deficits in attention, motor control and perception in 1975. Not until much later was I struck by the fact that some people I had met already in my own childhood must have been suffering from this disorder. Since 1985, Asperger syndrome and high-functioning autism have had a prominent place in my research. Over the years, I have personally followed several hundred children, adolescents and adults with Asperger syndrome. Some of these I have known and worked with closely for 20 years or more. At a more superficial level I have met many, many more with Asperger's particular variant of high-functioning autism.

All these unique human beings, with a common core nucleus of problems/personality features, are the backbone of this book. People with Asperger syndrome – with their lack of flexibility and, often, stunning egocentricity – have major problems coping with 'normal' life. At the same time, many are 'free thinkers' and may be scientifically or aesthetically highly skilled people. 'Asperger people' (as they sometimes like to refer to themselves) are fascinating and, possibly, specifically valuable for the development of the human species. Their difficulties and strengths shed light on the development and minds of other, 'neurotypical' (as those with Asperger syndrome sometimes refer to those who consider themselves 'normal') people.

Concluding remarks

It is almost 75 years since a Russian neurologist 'scientific assistant' described the syndrome that currently bears Hans Asperger's name. It is only in the past decade that Asperger syndrome has become recognised as one of the most important diagnostic categories in the whole of psychiatry.

Definitions

A diagnosis of Asperger syndrome cannot currently be made with confidence before the child's fifth birthday, and usually not until well into school age. This is partly because symptoms during the first few years may be subtle or uncharacteristic, partly because other diagnoses (including autistic disorder, ADHD and DAMP) may have been made and the 'Asperger problems' overlooked. The early symptoms are often sleep problems, 'stubbornness', passivity, attention problems, and unusual development of voice, speech and/or language.

This chapter deals with the definition of Asperger syndrome, and of other diagnostic concepts that will be repeatedly referred to in the book.

Asperger syndrome

Several years later, the *International Classification of Diseases* (ICD-10) published by WHO, included Asperger syndrome as a formal diagnosis for the first time (Table 2.3).

There are currently at least four definitions of Asperger syndrome that are frequently cited in the literature. Hans Asperger never published any formal diagnostic criteria. Lorna Wing, in her seminal 1981 paper, listed a number of symptoms but provided no algorithm for a final diagnosis.

The first operationalised diagnostic criteria to be presented were those of I. Carina Gillberg and Christopher Gillberg at the First International Conference on Asperger syndrome in London in 1988. These criteria were published in a scientific journal in 1989 and elaborated by Christopher Gillberg in 1991 (see Table 2.1). The six criteria are based on Asperger's descriptions of his first four published cases (Fritz, Harro, Ernst and Hellmuth from his 1944 paper). They underscore the importance of

Table 2.1 Diagnostic criteria for Asperger syndrome (according to Gillberg)

1. Social impairment (extreme egocentricity) (at least two of the following):
- (a) difficulties interacting with peers
- (b) indifference to peer contacts
- (c) difficulties interpreting social cues
- (d) socially and emotionally inappropriate behaviour

2. Narrow interest (at least one of the following):
- (a) exclusion of other activities
- (b) repetitive adherence
- (c) more rote than meaning

3. Compulsive need for introducing routines and interests (at least one of the following):
- (a) which affect the individual's every aspect of everyday life
- (b) which affect others

4. Speech and language peculiarities (at least three of the following):
- (a) delayed speech development
- (b) superficially perfect expressive language
- (c) formal pedantic language
- (d) odd prosody, peculiar voice characteristics
- (e) impairment of comprehension including misinterpretations of literal/implied meanings

5. Non-verbal communication problems (at least one of the following):
- (a) limited use of gestures
- (b) clumsy/gauche body language
- (c) limited facial expression
- (d) inappropriate facial expression
- (e) peculiar, stiff gaze

6. Motor clumsiness
poor performance in neurodevelopmental test

Source: Gillberg and Gillberg 1989, Gillberg 1991.

extreme egocentricity and major social interaction problems on the one hand, and the view, held by Asperger, that narrow interest patterns and motor clumsiness are crucial components of the condition, on the other. In line with Asperger's descriptions, they also include references to peculiarities of speech and language, in particular formalism and pedantic speech. When these criteria are used in research, all six have to be fulfilled for a definitive diagnosis to be made (and a total of 9 out of the 20 specified symptoms have to be met). In clinical practice, a diagnosis of Asperger syndrome is made if the social interaction dysfunction criterion is met along with at least four of the five other criteria.

Peter Szatmari published his four criteria in 1989 (Szatmari et al. 1989, 2000) (see Table 2.2). They resemble those of Gillberg and Gillberg (1989) to a considerable degree. However, Szatmari's diagnosis of Asperger syndrome can only be made if the individual does not meet criteria for autistic disorder. All four criteria have to be met (and a total of 6 out of the 22 specified symptoms).

Several years later, the *International Classification of Diseases and Disorders* (ICD-10) published by the WHO (1993), included Asperger syndrome as a formal diagnosis for the first time (Table 2.3). There is a strong emphasis on normal language and social development (as manifested by normal curiosity about the environment) in the first three years of life. The diagnosis cannot be made if criteria for childhood autism are (or were ever) met. Only eight symptoms are listed and a diagnosis requires that three of these be met.

The *Diagnostic and Statistical Manual of Mental Disorders* (DSM-IV) published by the American Psychiatric Association referred to 'Asperger's disorder' for the first time in 1994 (Table 2.4). The criteria are almost identical to those of the ICD-10. However, there is an important additional requirement of clinically significant impairment of functioning in work, socially or in other important aspects of life.

All of the four definitions are currently in use in the scientific study of Asperger syndrome. However, there are problems with all of them. Gillberg and Gillberg (1989) – in accordance with Hans Asperger's own view – require the presence of narrow interest patterns. Some individuals, girls and women in particular – while otherwise meeting all the criteria – do not show such interest patterns. Gillberg and Gillberg also require motor clumsiness for a definite diagnosis. Some people with otherwise classical Asperger symptoms have excellent motor skills. How should such individuals be diagnosed? In clinical practice, this is not a major problem given that 'only' five of the six criteria have to be met for a diagnosis to be made (see above). The Gillberg and Gillberg criteria can also be problematic in that the diagnosis can be made even when the algorithm for autistic disorder/

Table 2.2 Diagnostic criteria for Asperger syndrome (according to Szatmari)

---

1. Social isolation (at least two of the following):
   (a) no close friends
   (b) avoids others
   (c) no interest in making friends
   (d) a loner

2. Impaired social interaction (at least one of the following):
   (a) approaches others only to have own needs met
   (b) clumsy social approach
   (c) one-sided responses to peers
   (d) difficulty sensing feelings of others
   (e) indifference to the feelings of others

3. Impaired non-verbal communication (at least one of the following):
   (a) limited facial expression
   (b) impossible to read emotions through facial expression of the child
   (c) inability to convey message with eyes
   (d) avoids looking at others
   (e) does not use hands to aid expression
   (f) large and clumsy gestures
   (g) infringes on others people's physical space

4. Speech and language peculiarities (at least two of the following):
   (a) abnormalities of inflection
   (b) over-talkative
   (c) non-communicative
   (d) lack of cohesion to conversation
   (e) idiosyncratic use of words
   (f) repetitive patterns of speech

Source: Szatmari et al. (1989).

childhood autism is fulfilled. A recent study of high-functioning individuals in the autism spectrum showed many of those with 'Gillberg's' Asperger syndrome also met criteria for childhood autism. In clinical practice, a decision has to be made on which diagnosis is the one better accepted by the person affected and by parents or other carers. Currently, it seems to me that Asperger syndrome is often preferred over autism in cases meeting both sets of diagnostic criteria. Autism still has a 'pessimistic' ring to it, whereas Asperger syndrome, to many, does not carry equally negative

Table 2.3 Diagnostic criteria for Asperger syndrome (according to ICD-10)

1. There is no clinically significant general delay in spoken or receptive language or cognitive development

Diagnosis requires that single words should have developed by 2 years of age or earlier and that communicative phrases be used by 3 years of age or earlier. Self-help skills, adaptive behaviour, and curiosity about the environment during the first three years should be at a level consistent with normal intellectual development. However, motor milestones may be somewhat delayed and motor clumsiness is usual (although not a necessary diagnostic feature). Isolated special skills, often related to abnormal preoccupations, are common, but are not required for diagnosis.

2. There are qualitative abnormalities in reciprocal social interaction (in at least two of the following areas):

(a) failure adequately to use eye-to-eye gaze, facial expression, body posture and gesture to regulate social interaction

(b) failure to develop (in a manner appropriate to mental age, and despite ample opportunities) peer relationships that involve a mutual sharing of interests, activities and emotions

(c) lack of social–emotional reciprocity as shown by an impaired or deviant response to other people's emotions, or lack of modulation of behaviour according to social context; or a weak integration of social, emotional and communicative behaviours

(d) lack of spontaneous seeking to share enjoyment, interests or achievements with other people (e.g. lack of showing, bringing or pointing out to other people objects of interest to the individual)

3. The individual exhibits an unusually intense, circumscribed interest or restricted, repetitive and stereotyped patterns of behaviour, interests and activities (in at least two of the following):

(a) an encompassing preoccupation with one or more stereotyped and restricted patterns of interest that are abnormal in their intensity and circumscribed nature though not in their content or focus

(b) apparent compulsive adherence to specific, non-functional routines or rituals

(c) stereotyped and repetitive motor mannerisms that involve either hand- or finger-flapping or twisting, or complex whole-body movements

(d) preoccupations with part-objects or non-functional elements of play materials (such as their odour, the feel of their surface, or the noise or vibration that they generate

Source: WHO (1993).

Table 2.4 Diagnostic criteria for Asperger syndrome (acording to DSM-IV)

1. Qualitative impairment in social interaction (as manifested by at least two of the following):
  (a) marked impairment in the use of multiple non-verbal behaviours such as eye-to-eye gaze, facial expression, body postures and gesture to regulate social interaction
  (b) failure to develop peer relationships appropriate to developmental level
  (c) a lack of spontaneous seeking to share enjoyment, interests, or achievements with other people (e.g. by a lack of showing, bringing or pointing out objects of interest to other people)
  (d) lack of social or emotional reciprocity

2. Restricted or repetitive and stereotyped patterns of behaviour, interests and activities (as manifested by at least one of the following):
  (a) encompassing preoccupation with one or more stereotyped and restricted patterns of interest that is abnormal either in intensity or focus
  (b) apparently inflexible adherence to specific, non-functional routines or rituals
  (c) stereotyped and repetitive motor mannerisms (e.g. hand- or finger-flapping or twisting, or complex whole-body movements
  (d) persistent preoccupation with parts of objects

3. The disturbance causes clinically significant impairment in social, occupational or other important areas of functioning

4. There is no clinically significant general delay in language (e.g. single words used by age 2 years, communicative phrases used by age 3 years)

5. There is no clinically significant delay in cognitive development or in the development of age-appropriate self-help skills, adaptive behaviour (other than in social interaction), and curiosity about the environment in childhood

6. Criteria are not met for another specific developmental disorder or schizophrenia

Source: APA (1994).

connotations. This may change in the future, once it becomes generally accepted that autism spectrum disorders are not extremely rare, and that high-functioning cases, contrary to earlier beliefs, by far outnumber those that are very severely affected and low functioning.

Szatmari's criteria exclude a diagnosis of Asperger syndrome if autistic disorder criteria are met. However, clinical realities are such that individuals presenting with the problem constellation described by Asperger, very often meet criteria for autistic disorder or have met such criteria in the past. In fact, a study in which experts reviewed case histories without prior knowledge of who had written them up or which diagnoses had been made, showed all of Asperger's original cases met criteria for autistic disorder according to the DSM-IV.

This problem pertains to the DSM-IV and ICD-10 also. However, these manuals also cause major problems in that they include the criterion about normal development in the first three years of life. A study of 200 relatively high-functioning individuals with autism spectrum disorders, about half of whom had the 'classical' clinical presentation of Asperger syndrome, found only three who met the ICD-10 criteria for Asperger syndrome. This was because there are very few, if any, cases with the clinical symptoms of Asperger syndrome who have quite normal cognitive, language and social development in the first three years of life. The ICD-10 and DSM-IV are also problematic in that only three symptoms (out of the total of eight listed items) are required for diagnosis. This means that, from the symptomatic point of view, very little is required for a diagnosis of disorder to be made. Some children with depression, conduct disorder, exaggerated shyness or selective mutism actually have 'enough symptoms' to fit the diagnostic symptom criteria for Asperger syndrome of the ICD-10 (or the DSM-IV).

From now on, in this book, unless otherwise specified, the term Asperger syndrome will be used to refer to the variant described by Gillberg and Gillberg (1989).

Autism

The classic variant of autism described by Leo Kanner comprises a period of 'autistic aloneness' in infancy and 'insistence on sameness/elaborate repetitive routines'. Kanner's particular variant of autism appears to be only a rather narrow segment of the diagnostic category of autistic disorder/ childhood autism as outlined in the DSM-IV/ICD-10. All individuals meeting criteria for autistic disorder show the full triad of symptoms as described below under the heading of 'autism spectrum disorders', with marked problems of social reciprocity, communication and behaviour and/or imagination.

Cases with autism can be grouped into those that are 'low-functioning', 'middle-functioning' and 'high-functioning'. In the latter group, IQ is usually in the low normal or normal range. It is this subgroup of those with autistic disorder that causes the most debate when it comes to the diagnosis of Asperger syndrome. Some authors maintain the position that it would be more reasonable to refer those currently diagnosed as having Asperger syndrome to the category of high-functioning autism (HFA). Others are of the opinion that Asperger syndrome is a helpful concept in that it is more 'neutral' than terms including reference to autism, and that the word 'autism' has too many negative connotations. Given that the majority of individuals showing the clinical picture of Asperger syndrome are *very* high functioning, they certainly differ enormously from those with low-functioning autism. To be able to use two different terms for clinical conditions that are so different – in spite of probably belonging in the same general category of 'autism spectrum disorders' – is helpful.

Autism spectrum disorders

The term autism spectrum disorders is used here to cover all syndromes comprising major functional impairments in at least two of the three areas: (1) reciprocal social interaction; (2) reciprocal verbal and non-verbal communication; and (3) imagination and behaviour. When all three areas are affected, the term 'Lorna Wing's triad' is often used. Wing, in the 1970s, found that the combination of these three symptoms was what is common to all individuals diagnosed as having childhood autism (Wing 1981).

The umbrella concept of autism spectrum disorders (broadly synonymous with the concept of 'pervasive developmental disorders') comprises autistic disorder (also referred to as Kanner syndrome, infantile autism, childhood autism, or just simply 'autism'), Asperger syndrome, childhood disintegrative disorder (CDD) and other autistic-like conditions (see Table 2.5). Some authorities would also include autistic features and 'the broader autism phenotype'/'the lesser variant of autism' (see below, p. 13).

There are also those who use the term 'autism spectrum disorders' differently, and apply it only in cases with autistic-like conditions that do not meet the full criteria for autistic disorder/childhood autism.

Some authors also use the term 'autistic continuum' to indicate that there is a range of autistic conditions with 'severe' cases at one end and

Table 2.5 Autism spectrum disorders – synonyms

Autism
     Kanner syndrome
     Autistic disorder
     Childhood autism
     Infantile autism

Asperger syndrome
     Asperger's disorder
     Autistic psychopathy
     (High-functioning autism?)

Childhood disintegrative disorder
     Heller syndrome
     Dementia infantilis

Other autistic-like conditions
     Atypical autism
     Pervasive developmental disorder not otherwise specified (PDD NOS)

The lesser variant of autism
     Broader phenotype of autism
     (Autistic features/DAMP with autistic features)

'mild' cases at the other. This term seems to me to be less useful. It presupposes that all autistic and autistic-like conditions can be grouped according to severity along a continuum. In some individuals with Asperger syndrome the condition is actually very severe, more severe than 'a mild case of autistic disorder'. Yet, within the continuum framework, Asperger syndrome would generally be classified as a 'milder' condition than autistic disorder, which, in turn, would be considered 'severe'.

The broader phenotype (lesser variant) of autism

Recent genetic studies of autism have demonstrated that a 'lesser variant' of the condition often exists in relatives of those affected by severe disorders. This 'broader phenotype' can show as mild autistic-type symptoms (for instance, as social withdrawal, shyness, mild social phobia, inflexible and stilted language, obsessive-compulsive phenomena and rigid behaviours), even when there is no major functional clinical impairment and the condition cannot be regarded as handicapping.

Non-verbal learning difficulties

The concept of non-verbal learning difficulties has been developed by neuropsychologists. Interest in this category has grown alongside the emerging interest in the syndrome that Asperger described. It refers to a combination of problems that share many features with Asperger syndrome: difficulties in procedural learning, visuospatial dysfunction, social interaction problems and peculiarities of intonation, but no abnormalities of formal spoken language. It is likely that some individuals with a diagnosis of non-verbal learning difficulty would have received a diagnosis of Asperger syndrome 'instead' had he/she consulted a psychiatrist with expertise in autism spectrum disorders. Non-verbal learning difficulties are believed to be associated with reduced function in the right cerebral hemisphere (see chapter 10).

Semantic–pragmatic disorder

Children and adults with Asperger syndrome have major problems with pragmatics even while usually exhibiting excellent expressive language skills. While having a large vocabulary and perfect knowledge of the meaning of individual words, they often have great difficulty using these words in everyday life for two-way interactive communication. They also fail to keep a conversation going and may not understand or react to verbal approaches made by other people. Their prosody is very often odd and their level and tone of voice unusual or abnormal.

All or most of these problems are also encountered in individuals with 'semantic-pragmatic disorder'. This is a concept developed by speech and language experts, linguists and neurologists. As with non-verbal learning difficulty, it is likely that many if not all people diagnosed with this condition would also meet criteria for Asperger syndrome or another autism spectrum disorder. Right-hemisphere brain dysfunction has been proposed to underlie this combination of problems. The borderlands of Asperger syndrome, non-verbal learning difficulties, 'right-hemisphere dysfunction' and semantic-pragmatic disorder clearly overlap. It is possible that they are all related to the field of autism spectrum disorders.

It is unclear, at the present stage, to what extent people with Asperger syndrome have any 'semantic problems'. The children I have seen who have been diagnosed by other experts as having semantic-pragmatic disorder did not have obvious semantic problems but major, severely handicapping, pragmatic problems.

Attention-deficit/hyperactivity disorder

A considerable proportion of all children in the general population has attention-deficit/hyperactivity disorder (ADHD). Most studies suggest that the rate of clinically significant disorder is at least in the order of 3%, with boys outnumbering girls by at least two to one. ADHD usually presents with severe attentional deficits during the first year of life and with continuing problems throughout the preschool years. Some children are severely – and chronically – hyperactive, but the majority are not, fluctuating between hypo-activity and mild-moderate hyperactivity. Impulsivity is also usually, but certainly not invariably, part of the picture.

ADHD is diagnosed in accordance with the DSM-IV on the basis of a minimum of either (i) six symptoms (out of nine possible) of inattention; (ii) six symptoms (out of nine possible) of hyperactivity-impulsivity; or (iii) both six inattention and six hyperactivity symptoms. The three subtypes are labelled (i) ADHD – mainly inattentive; (ii) ADHD – mainly hyperactive-impulsive; and (iii) ADHD – combined.

Many individuals with Asperger syndrome and other autistic-like conditions show severe degrees of inattention and impulsivity and many meet the symptom criteria for ADHD of the DSM-IV.

It is important to consider the possibility of ADHD in Asperger syndrome. There are a number of very helpful interventions that need to be considered in cases with severe inattention/hyperactivity. Some clinicians feel that a diagnosis of Asperger syndrome is 'sufficient' and that making additional comorbid diagnoses is not appropriate. However, long-term clinical experience suggests that the major attentional and activity problems shown by so many individuals with autism spectrum disorder need to be taken into account and treated in their own right.

Developmental coordination disorder (DCD)

Motor clumsiness can affect gross motor activities as well as fine motor functions. Regardless, when problems are severe and interfere with everyday activities, a diagnosis of developmental coordination disorder (DCD) should be made. About 5% of children in the general population have a marked variant of DCD. Moderate and mild problems in this area are much more common and affect about 1 in 10 of all individuals.

Children, and adults, with Asperger syndrome always have some motor problems, at least according to the research criteria set out by Gillberg and Gillberg (1989). Asperger himself considered motor control problems to be very important in autistic psychopathy. Conversely, children with DCD are often socially impaired.

The common comorbidity of motor control problems and social interaction difficulties makes it imperative to try and work up both types of problems in children presenting with developmental difficulties.

Deficits in attention, motor control and perception (DAMP)

In Scandinavia, the concept of DAMP ('deficits in attention, motor control and perception') has become rooted over the past 20 years. Interest in the concept has grown considerably in recent years, and it is now a diagnosis that is widely discussed in the United Kingdom, Australasia and the United States also.

The diagnosis refers to syndromes in which children (or adults) show the combination of ADHD and DCD. About 2% of the general population of children starting school meet criteria for severe DAMP, and another 3% or so have moderate problems. The syndrome is overrepresented in boys.

Clinical experience, and several empirical studies, have shown that DAMP is very often on a continuum with autism spectrum disorders. Any child meeting criteria for DAMP is much more likely than other children to have social interaction problems. Conversely, individuals with social interaction problems on the autism spectrum very often have motor control and attentional problems.

One study suggested that if an individual receives a diagnosis of Asperger syndrome, the likelihood that he/she will also fulfil criteria for DAMP is very high. Thus, any manual suggesting that an autism spectrum disorder diagnosis or an ADHD/DCD diagnosis should exclude a diagnosis of any problem within the autism spectrum, needs to be regarded with great caution.

Tourette syndrome

Tics of different kinds are common in children, adolescents and adults with autism spectrum disorders. In Asperger syndrome they may be particularly frequent (affecting up to 80% according to one study). They also occur very often in the general population, affecting at least 1 in 10 of all school-age children at one point in time or another. Tics can affect peripheral muscles and be termed 'motor' or be vocal phenomena leading to the production of compulsive spasmodic sounds, words or sentences.

Tourette syndrome, which affects about 1% of the school age population of children (boys, again, being much more often affected than girls), is diagnosed on the basis of the presence of multiple motor and one or more vocal tics, in individuals clinically impaired by their tics. Tourette syndrome occurs in a percentage of children with classic autism and possibly in as many as one in five in Asperger syndrome.

Obsessive–compulsive disorder (OCD)

Rigid, repetitive, pedantic, perfectionist, obsessive and compulsive phenomena are part and parcel of virtually all autism spectrum disorders, including Asperger syndrome. There is sometimes a problem distinguishing obsessive–compulsive disorder as a diagnosis separate from the autism spectrum disorder. This is particularly the case when the individual feels that the obsessions and compulsions are normal phenomena and an integral part of the personality. Nevertheless, in cases with Asperger syndrome and other disorders in the autism spectrum, whenever obsessions, compulsions, ritualistic phenomena or insistence on sameness are so incapacitating as to warrant specific intervention, a separate diagnosis of comorbid OCD should be made.

About 1% of children and adolescents in the general population have incapacitating symptoms of OCD. Boys and girls are about equally affected.

Table 2.6 Diagnostic criteria for obsessive–compulsive personality disorder (DSM-IV)

A pervasive pattern of preoccupation with orderliness, perfectionism and mental and interpersonal control, at the expense of flexibility, openness and efficiency, beginning by early adulthood and present in a variety of contexts (as indicated by at least four of the following):

(1) is preoccupied with details, rules, lists, order, organisation or schedules to the extent that the major point of the activity is lost

(2) shows perfectionism that interferes with task completion (e.g. is unable to complete a project because his or her own overly strict standards are not met)

(3) is excessively devoted to work and productivity to the exclusion of leisure activities and friendships (not accounted for by obvious economic necessity)

(4) is overconscientious, scrupulous and inflexible about matters of morality, ethics or values (not accounted for by cultural or religious identification)

(5) is unable to discard worn-out or worthless objects even when they have no sentimental value

(6) is reluctant to delegate tasks or to work with others unless they submit to exactly his or her way of doing things

(7) adopts a miserly spending style towards both self and others; money is viewed as something to be hoarded for future catastrophes

(8) shows rigidity and stubbornness

Source: APA (1994).

Obsessive–compulsive personality disorder (OCPD) is conceptualised as a chronic personality disorder in which obsessions and compulsions are prominent (Table 2.6). If one looks closely at the DSM-IV criteria for this disorder, one is struck by the general similarity of this diagnostic concept and that of Asperger syndrome. It is currently unclear whether there are any distinct boundaries between OCPD and Asperger syndrome.

Conduct disorder and oppositional defiant disorder (ODD)

The hallmarks of conduct disorder and oppositional-defiant disorder (ODD) are social interaction problems, including socially unacceptable, aggressive and destructive behaviours. Children given these diagnoses are oppositional, verbally abusive, negativistic, complaining and protesting. In conduct disorder there are also activities which are clearly transgressive of societal norms, and many commit acts that are considered to be criminal and would have been judged as such had the individual been over the age of 16 or 18 years. By tradition, conduct disorder (listed in both ICD-10 and DSM-IV) and ODD (not included in the ICD classification system, but a coveted term in the DSM manual), have come to be regarded as very much unlike Asperger syndrome and other autistic-like conditions. Nevertheless, people with conduct disorder often display the same kind of empathy problems that are believed to be at the core of Asperger syndrome. Oppositional and defiant behaviours are also common in Asperger syndrome. The boundaries between autism spectrum disorders and conduct disorder/ODD are, by no means clear. Conduct disorder as a 'psychiatric' diagnosis rather than a descriptive term for a particular kind of unacceptable behaviour is also debatable. There is a clear need for more research when it comes to the relationship between autism spectrum disorders and conduct problems both in children/adolescents and adults.

ODD is a common associated diagnosis in ADHD (and DAMP). It is very likely that had a diagnosis of ODD been considered in cases with autism spectrum disorders, it would have become clear that ODD behaviours are extremely common in Asperger syndrome and other high-functioning disorders in the autism spectrum.

Concluding remarks

At least four different diagnostic systems for Asperger syndrome are currently in use. Of these, those of the ICD-10 and the DSM-IV are closely similar, but also very problematic in that few, if any, individuals with the classical presentation of Asperger syndrome (as described by Hans Asperger) fit their diagnostic criteria. The criteria of Szatmari (1989) and of Gillberg and Gillberg (1989) provide much more detailed accounts of the clinical picture. This book will mostly refer to the Gillberg criteria.

There are very few – if any – conditions that cannot – and do not – exist together with autism spectrum disorders. ADHD/DAMP, tics and Tourette syndrome, OCD/OCPD and conduct disorder/ODD can all cause considerable differential diagnostic controversy. The 'take-home' message is that Asperger syndrome, high-functioning autism and other autistic-like conditions can, and do, exist alongside any other disorder.

Prevalence

Population studies

The rate at which Asperger syndrome occurs in the general population has only been the subject of a few studies, the majority of which have been concerned with school-age children and performed in the Nordic countries. Therefore, it is difficult at the present stage to draw any generalised conclusions about the prevalence of the syndrome. It is impossible to determine whether or not Asperger syndrome is equally common across the globe, and, even, whether or not it occurs in all countries.

The first population study of the occurrence of Asperger syndrome was performed in Göteborg, Sweden in the early 1980s. About 5,000 children born in 1971 were screened and followed up in intensive neuropsychiatric studies. A minimum rate of 26 in 10,000 children was ascertained for 'Asperger syndrome' as described by Gillberg (1991). The rate of 'disorder' was similar if ICD-10 criteria were used and the requirement of normal development in the first three years of life disregarded. The focus of the study was on ADHD and DAMP (see chapter 2) and so the prevalence of Asperger syndrome must be regarded as a rough estimate.

More reliable estimates of disorder were obtained in two later studies specifically geared at evaluating prevalence rates of the disorder in school-age children. In a study performed in Göteborg in 1992, the rate of 'typical' Asperger syndrome (Gillberg and Gillberg criteria) in school-age children (7–16 years of age) was estimated at 36 in 10,000 children. Another 36 in 10,000 had autism spectrum disorders similar to Asperger syndrome, but not meeting full research criteria for the disorder, or for classic autism. If the criterion of normal development in the first three years of life was disregarded, the children meeting Gillberg criteria also met ICD-10 criteria for

Asperger syndrome. This population prevalence estimate must be regarded as very rough and in need of replication by other groups. The so-called 95% confidence interval – a measure of the accuracy of the estimate – ranged from 11 though 84 in 10,000 children. In another small-scale Swedish study, performed in 1998, the rate of Asperger syndrome was 48 in 10,000 children (11-year-olds) (Kadesjö, Gillberg and Hagberg 1999). A study from Iceland in the early 1980s corroborated the findings from the Swedish studies, reporting a prevalence rate of 35 in 10,000 individuals of school age. Somewhat higher estimates were recently published by a Baltic group (Lesinskiene and Puras 2001). Two recent British studies have found rates of 'autism spectrum disorders'/'pervasive developmental disorders' (encompassing both autistic disorder, and Asperger syndrome) that are broadly consistent with those of the Nordic studies (see Chakrabarti and Fombonne 2001). The 'exact' rate of Asperger syndrome is, of course, heavily dependent on the diagnostic criteria used, and since there is currently no consensus in this respect, reported rates cannot be expected to be identical across studies. Some authors would use the term 'autism spectrum disorder' when others refer to 'Asperger syndrome'. This means that estimates of the prevalence of Asperger syndrome will have to take reports on autism spectrum disorder into account (and vice versa).

Clinic-based studies

In clinic-based studies, the rate of Asperger syndrome has tended to be much higher, depending also on the type of clinic involved in the study. Child psychiatric clinic attenders have been reported to have Asperger syndrome in about 5% of all cases. Interestingly, the Swedish studies suggest that only about half of all classic Asperger syndrome cases get referred to child and adolescent psychiatrists. Some classic cases are assessed by child neurologists or developmental paediatricians. Others still apply for help only in adult age, at a time when it is likely that their problems will be misunderstood and diagnosis may be further delayed or inappropriate. A percentage of all adult psychiatric outpatients diagnosed as having psychosis, obsessive–compulsive disorders or personality disorders were shown to have Asperger syndrome and other autism spectrum disorders in a recent study from the south of Sweden (Nylander and Gillberg 2001).

The frequency of Asperger syndrome in young adults who have committed severe and violent crimes appears to be raised above the level of occurrence in the general population. However, this is certainly not to say that people with Asperger syndrome often commit serious crimes. On the contrary, the vast majority of those with the syndrome are law-abiding citizens and are strongly opposed to any kind of violence.

Male versus female ratios

The ratio of boys to girls in Asperger syndrome is raised much above that in the general population. Most studies suggest that the proportion is in the order of three to six males to every female with the syndrome.

Girls and women with Asperger syndrome sometimes show a slightly different constellation of symptoms than the one regarded as typical of males with the disorder (see also chapter 4). It is quite conceivable that such cases would be missed in epidemiological studies. This, in turn, infers that current prevalence figures are underestimates, and that the proportion of females with the condition is larger than usually reported.

Concluding remarks

Probably about 3–4 in every 1,000 children develop the full clinical picture of Asperger syndrome before about 10 years of age. A similar proportion of the general population has other autism spectrum disorders that only just fail to meet full criteria for Asperger syndrome. Males have the typical symptoms much more often than females, and only about one in five classical cases is female. The diagnosis is currently overlooked in some girls with core deficits but without the typical 'male interest patterns'. Only about half of all children affected actually apply for child and adolescent psychiatric help. Many of these, and probably several more, apply for psychiatric help in adult age, but the diagnosis of Asperger syndrome is often missed in this latter group of cases.

Symptoms in childhood

Asperger syndrome is usually congenital or arises on the basis of brain damage sustained during parturition or the first few years of life. Very rarely does it appear as a consequence of brain damage acquired later in life. It is common for symptoms not to become conspicuous until the child's fourth year or even later, and diagnosis is often not made until well into the school years.

In retrospect, it is often possible to get convincing descriptions of symptoms that were present already in the first two years of life. For the most part, these symptoms are subtle as compared with the rather more obvious problems encountered in classic autism. In a subgroup there is evidence of major social and communication deficits already in the first year of life. A diagnosis of autism may have been discussed or actually made in such cases. In yet other cases there is little or no evidence of symptoms before the child's third year. The symptoms that then emerge are often vague – or vaguely perceived/described – and the diagnosis rarely considered, much less made, in the early years.

It is not uncommon for children who are later diagnosed as having Asperger syndrome to have an early development reminiscent of or virtually identical to that seen in children with ADHD or DAMP (see chapter 2). There is a great degree of symptomatic overlap between cases with Asperger syndrome and cases with severe DAMP.

Some individuals have early onset overactivity, lack of impulse control and attention deficits, often in combination with severe sleep disturbance. A diagnosis of ADHD may have been considered or already made. A few years later, around age 3–5 years, there may be concerns regarding language, balance and motor incoordination, and the diagnosis may be 'changed' to DAMP. Around age 6–8 years, it may become obvious that problems with reciprocal social interaction may be those that overshadow the other symptoms and represent the most marked deviance from so-called normality. To the diagnosis of DAMP may be added that of 'autistic features'. Many years later, when the affected individual applies for adult psychiatric help, Asperger syndrome may be the only diagnosis considered by the young, recently trained psychiatrist.

In other cases, development seems to take the opposite direction. Major autistic symptoms appear early in the life of the child with gaze avoidance, poor attention, panic and confusion states, refusal to be comforted and marked delay in all social and communicative domains. A diagnosis of autism may actually have been made before the child's fourth birthday. During the early school years, the clinical presentation may have changed to the extent that classic Asperger syndrome is the only 'reasonable' clinical diagnosis. In early adolescence, a diagnosis of DAMP may seem the most appropriate for the doctor or psychologist who never met the patient when he/she was very young. In early adulthood, affected individuals may be considered 'normal' with only some oddities of personal style, an eccentric mode of communication and a certain motor clumsiness or 'motor peculiarity'.

In the majority of such cases, in which diagnoses seem to blend or merge into one another, one is, of course, dealing with chronic functional impairments with a common core but with variable symptom presentation over the years. Occasionally, it is a matter of distinct conditions occurring together either by coincidence or for reasons that are not coincidental. In the latter case it could be a matter of dysfunction/damage hitting the brain at distinctly different locations or functional loops during the last third of intrauterine life.

The first two years

There are no symptoms in the first years of life that should alert a parent or clinician to the possibility of Asperger syndrome. Not enough is yet known about the very early symptoms of the disorder to warrant any kind of screening for the disorder in infancy. However, some classic symptoms of autism may be present very early, but it is not possible at this early stage of development to determine whether or not the clinical picture will later be one of low-, middle- or high-functioning autism or more clearly compatible with the features described by Asperger. There are commonly unspecific indications that development may not be quite normal, and there are often problems that could signal any neurodevelopmental or neuropsychiatric disorder or just be transient symptoms that are common in children who do not later exhibit marked problems of any kind.

Many individuals who later present with the classical clinical picture of Asperger syndrome show such subtle symptoms or signs in early life that parents and other people close to the family do not suspect a serious problem of any kind.

Unspecific symptoms

Abnormal sleep patterns, poor attention (perhaps particularly poor auditory attention), overactivity or extreme passivity, poor bodily adaptability (such as the child failing to adjust in the mother's arms when feeding), staring gaze and fixation on detail appear to be overrepresented in Asperger syndrome and may be present from a very early age. A few children start walking long before their first birthday, others around the expected time (of about 11–13 months) whereas others still (quite a large group, see below) are late onset walkers.

Some are described as unusually good and easy during the first year of life, maybe with slightly delayed motor development but with early indications of good vocal and language imitation skills. Some seem to be particularly happy when left alone and when demands for attention are not made by other people.

Other children who later develop the classic picture of Asperger syndrome appear much more 'disturbed' already during the first year of life. They scream a lot, are difficult to comfort, fluctuate between extremes of hyperactivity and (more rarely) apathy, appear to be 'in pain' and may have marked sleep problems. ADHD may be considered in such children, and follow-up will sometimes show them to meet diagnostic criteria both for ADHD and Asperger syndrome (sometimes also for Tourette syndrome).

Classic autism symptoms

Judging from my own clinical experience, there are some common early symptoms of autism that can sometimes be encountered in children who later meet full diagnostic criteria for Asperger syndrome. These are unusual reactions to sensory stimuli (sound, smell and touch in particular), abnormalities of gaze behaviour (staring, less 'lively' than other children, 'big-eyed and lost', does not follow other people's gaze direction) and looking 'too old and wise'. It is quite common for pointing to appear later than in normal development, and particularly for pointing to indicate the need/ urge to share attention with other people. Severe social withdrawal is probably uncommon, even though there are certainly individuals who show so-called 'autistic aloneness' and 'stand-offish manner' before the age of 3 years.

Developmental problems

Even though the ICD and DSM manuals require normal early language development for a diagnosis of Asperger syndrome to be made, the majority of children with the condition do have some obvious or subtle abnormalities/delays in the development of spoken language and in the understanding of the meaning of communication. Language may develop later than in siblings or may be marked by unusual first words and a strong tendency to echolalia (repetition of words and phrases, including, in rare cases, verbatim recounting of whole sitcom episodes, poems or complicated song texts). It is not uncommon for the child to be able to imitate other people – and even foreign languages – from a very early age, in which case, 'language' is usually felt to be extremely advanced. Such imitation skills may mask underlying severe communication deficits. The child may make spontaneous 'comments' about things he/she sees or hears, but fails to respond to any questions or other approaches (by well-known people or strangers). Comprehension may be abnormal even though the understanding of single words appears to be (and may well be) unimpaired. It is not uncommon for children with Asperger syndrome to say nothing even when they would have had the actual skills to say something. A minority appear to have well-developed expressive language skills for months or even years before they start making use of them. This could be the case if a child says his first words at the age of four years, and they are: 'No thank you, I do not much like apples!' Many parents report that they believe their child could read well before he/she started talking. Hyperlexia can sometimes be corroborated at testing in such cases.

young age have developed extreme talents in areas such as computers, geography, mathematics or sports results. They may be perceived as leaders who try to involve other children in more or less destructive play. Superficially in such cases there may be the impression of friendship, even though closer analysis will reveal the lack of real social reciprocity.

Parents may be concerned about the child's lack of empathy. Devastated mothers have asked me if it is possible that their sons have no capacity for empathy at all. More commonly they worry about the child's lack of age peers. Some children actually try to 'comfort' their parents by asserting that they need not be worried by their lack of friends: 'I can do excellently without so-called friends. They are usually only dull, uninteresting creatures who I would not want to spend time with anyway. They only play their own stupid games. My interests are much more satisfying.' Similar phrases may be uttered by children with Asperger syndrome already around age 5 years, often in a distinctly articulated way almost as though reading aloud out of a book. Boys with Asperger syndrome are often good readers already at this young age. Their mechanical reading skills are usually much better developed than their ability to speak without impediment or to keep up even a simple conversation.

Spontaneous communicative speech – that is, utterances that do not appear to be mere rote memory phrases, clichés or outright echolalia – may be surprisingly limited, inarticulate or 'mumbling'.

The early school years

There are many children with Asperger syndrome who start school without anybody really suspecting that something might be seriously amiss. From about age 6 years to the late pre-adolescent years, the clinical picture usually becomes more striking, and it is during this time period that the features are often so characteristic that the diagnosis is rarely missed if it is considered. While the syndrome that Kanner described is usually most characteristic in the preschool years – and therefore diagnosed during that period – Asperger syndrome is almost never diagnosed until the early school years.

All the characteristic symptoms are usually represented around age 8–10 years. The following section contains a 'symptom by symptom' account of classic Asperger syndrome as it presents in this age group.

Markedly reduced capacity for social reciprocity

This symptom is often perceived as 'extreme egocentricity'. This, in turn, is usually a catchphrase for the reduced capacity to go beyond the limits of 'the self' and to take the cognitive or emotional perspectives of other people. The child will behave in emotionally and socially inappropriate ways. There is often a mixture of precocious behaviours and social immaturity, and the child's overall approach in communication with other people may be regarded either as provocative or extremely naive. An almost pathological need to always tell the truth is striking in many cases. The child does not appear to understand 'self-evident' social rules, and cannot be persuaded to keeping his thoughts ('truths') to him/herself. The teacher at school may be told that she has a foul breath, is ignorant, or that she has ill-fitting clothes. Alternatively, she may be 'complimented' on having such a nice bra. All of these things may well be 'true'. The problem is that the child with Asperger syndrome does not understand social rules, cannot judge the situation, and is unable to conclude that 'certain things you just do not say in certain settings'. There will always be things that are socially inappropriate in some situations or will be felt to be hurtful in any situation: the child with Asperger syndrome often appears to be 'blind' to such matters. Many completely refuse to abstain from always telling the truth, and will not ever 'play along' or 'act a role'. Others gradually develop a great skill for acting and manage to take on different (well-rehearsed) roles for different occasions, but often have difficulty 'keeping up appearances' over more than a very short period of time. Some 'take after' their brother, sister, class-mate, or an adult, and come across, at least to those who know them over a longer period, as 'social chameleons' ('Zelig syndrome'). On a one-to-one basis, however, such individuals quickly run out of material and there may be no more situation-appropriate roles to play. The basic impairment – the reduced ability to interact socially with a partner in an automatic, intuitive and 'quick' way – will then stand out as all the more dramatic.

The egocentricity usually makes it hard to find real friends. The majority of those with Asperger syndrome are not troubled by their lack of friends, at least not during the early school years. Gradually, many become aware of being 'odd', 'unusual' or 'different'. Some worry that they may not 'be normal'. Certain individuals with Asperger syndrome have an almost obsessive idea that people should be normal, although many, luckily, do not care about 'normality'. Those who are preoccupied with being normal often start saying that they would like to have friends during the pre-adolescent years. They may ask their parents to ring up a same-aged child and ask him over. They may think and talk a lot about the 'friend's coming over to play' and eagerly await his/her arrival. When finally the 'friend' appears, the child with Asperger syndrome seems to have forgotten all about that eagerness. He may not even look up from the book he is reading, a book he obviously finds infinitely more interesting than the 'friend'.

Some can be with other children, but not really in a turn-taking mutual, sharing fashion. Either they want to 'run the show', play in a parallel fashion, or, occasionally submit to another leader's rigid curriculum, without making any demands whatsoever. Many schoolchildren with Asperger syndrome are accepted much more unquestioningly by adults – and sometimes also by much younger children – than by age peers. Same-aged children make greater demands on acceptable social behaviours from those whom they want to play with, and they also themselves have greater difficulty adjusting to other people's needs. Younger children may 'look up to the little professor' or just become fascinated with all the knowledge shown by the child with Asperger syndrome. However, most school-age children with autism spectrum disorders have major difficulties interacting socially both with adults and with very young children.

The child with Asperger syndrome often refuses to go along with the demands made by adults. Particularly difficult situations may arise if the adult patiently tries to explain (perhaps in a convoluted way) what may be considered conventional wisdom or the underlying reason for a social tradition (such as why not *all* truths should be spelled out to *all* people one meets). The child then may start arguing and the adult may well find himself painted into a corner. The child will find constantly new arguments (albeit that they are variations on a repetitive theme), and the 'discussion' will only terminate after the adult has said (what he/she should perhaps have said all along): 'You simply do not do that!' Rather surprisingly, many individuals with Asperger syndrome will be better satisfied with such 'explanations' about social rules. On other occasions it may be a good investment of time to sit down and explain in detail, but only if the explanation starts on a very basic level. This is usually best done 'after the fact'. It is easier if the child is well aware of his/her own diagnosis, so that the adult can relate the explanation to the child's well-known difficulties.

Many people with Asperger syndrome lack common sense. Much of what governs our social interactions is intuitive, and something which is expected to be known almost without explicit training. It is difficult to define 'common sense'. Even so, most people, even school-age children have an inkling of what is inferred by the term. People with Asperger syndrome are so severely handicapped in this domain that they may themselves feel that they do not know 'how to live'. They appear lost and forlorn. It is usually only towards the end of the pre-adolescent period that it becomes obvious that individuals with Asperger syndrome are so totally lacking in common sense.

Narrow interest patterns

Very narrow interest patterns are often very conspicuous during the school years, and may develop into a major problem. Most of the time it is not the interest *content* that is problematic, but rather the *way* in which the child gets absorbed in the interest. It is important to distinguish between having a hobby/interest on the one hand and the kind of obsessive pursuit of narrow interests which is the rule in Asperger syndrome on the other.

Boys with Asperger syndrome often amass facts about certain aspects of the environment and learn them by heart. It could be to do with anything, but the possibility to record and list aspects of the interest appears to hold a special fascination. 'Top charts' are often produced out of the pockets of boys with Asperger syndrome, with lists of the 50 highest mountains, the 30 best jokes etc. Girls' interests may sometimes, at least superficially, appear to be more 'social', but, on further analysis, one often finds that they are also dependent on rote memory rather than meaning. Some girls (and a few boys) appear to have few or even no interests. They are often generally characterised by negativism and a tendency to say 'No' to just about everything. Some of these are similar to the children described by Elisabeth Newson (Newson and Newson 1983), and whom she refers to as 'pathological demand avoiders'.

Historical events, capitals of the world, meteorology, dinosaurs, archaeology, cinema and famous actors, opera singers, Chinese pottery, the French revolution, mathematics, prime numbers, Rommel's desert wars, mycology,

Austria during the second world war, female opera singers, tram timetables, the telephone directory, frogs, Cromwell, Sainsbury's, make-up, the gastro-intestinal system, dolls, computers, fish and chips, red Indians of North America, Rowan Atkinson and Björn Borg are only some of the special interests I and others who have listened have been allowed to share with school-age children with Asperger syndrome.

For an older person it can be quite rewarding, at least for a few minutes, to sit down and listen to the child's monologue. There is often a possibility that one might learn something, whether it is in an area inside or outside one's own area of expertise. Oftentimes it becomes tedious to have to listen to all the details. For instance, to have to listen to *all* the song-texts of Lennon–McCartney without being allowed to ask even a single question, can be too much even for a trained listener. Same-aged children can sometimes be impressed by all this knowledge shown by the child with Asperger syndrome, who can then be regarded as special, fantastic or a whiz-kid, and become the centre of everybody's attention. Much more commonly though, the opposite occurs, and the child with Asperger syndrome with his special interest is regarded as absurd, weird or crazy. This may then lead on to bullying activities which may either – at least not primarily – not be noted by the child with Asperger syndrome, or be the beginning of a terrible sequence of events that may lead to depression and suicide attempts.

The special interest is usually isolated in the sense that it does not inspire interest in other, neighbouring, areas. A 10-year-old boy with a special interest in the French queen Marie Antoinette, who knew all about her last years – and hence quite a lot of detail about the geography of Paris – did not himself remember that he already knew something about Paris when, later, the map of Paris became his number one interest. His father had to remind him that he in fact already knew the locations of La Conciergerie, L'Église de Notre Dame and La Bastille.

Sometimes there are two or three interests at the same time, but rarely more than that. The interests may come and go, even though a proportion will stick with their first 'and only' interest throughout life. Even when interests change, the style in which they are adhered to rarely does. Again, it has to be said that it is not the interest in itself, but rather the character of the person's relationship to the interest, that is the problem. The individual with Asperger syndrome so engrosses himself in the interest that it becomes tedious, indeed often painfully so, for other people. So much time, energy and thought are spent on it, that there is little or no time left for anything else.

Repetitive thoughts, actions, ritualism and dependence on routines

An almost obsessive desire to introduce routines and rituals of different kinds are the rule in Asperger syndrome and often become handicapping only in middle childhood. There is often a need to repeat thoughts and phrases 'inside the head' and to perform a variety of repetitive actions. Routines and rituals are often directly linked to special interests, but will also impose on other activities, such as dressing, feeding, watching television, transportation, or matters to do with personal hygiene. It is very common for other members of the family to be drawn into these 'ideas' and forced to 'abide by them', no matter how absurd they may seem. Sometimes, the child with Asperger syndrome 'makes himself perform' to perform a number of activities before he can start doing something else. Obsessions and compulsions can sometimes be so severe that separate symptom criteria for obsessive–compulsive disorder or obsessive–compulsive personality disorder are met. In certain cases, these obsessions and compulsions may need to be seen as a separate problem that may warrant specific treatment (pharmacotherapy, cognitive behaviour therapy or both).

Communication problems affecting speech and language

Speech and language are also usually affected in Asperger syndrome, in spite of the fact that the ICD-10 and DSM-IV include no reference to this in their diagnostic criteria. Most active researchers in the field acknowledge the existence of a number of speech and language peculiarities in Asperger syndrome. Many consider them to be a reflection of the core problems in the syndrome.

Some language delay is common in Asperger syndrome (see above), but during the school years there is usually no or little reflection of this in symptomatology. However, a proportion of school-age children with Asperger syndrome has some articulation problems, and there may be a 'childish ring' to speech, even when the language content may be 'overly adult'. Hyperlexia is common, meaning that mechanical reading skills may be excellent, even though comprehension may (or may not) be impaired. Language comprehension problems are common even in cases with excellent vocabulary. Children with Asperger syndrome may be masters of single words but still have difficulty understanding language *in context*. They may have problems with metaphoric language, or, indeed any language that has not been explicitly explained to them. It is not uncommon for them to misunderstand the intentions of other people. 'Could you open the door for me?' somebody might say, and the child with Asperger may respond 'Yes', but do nothing. She understood the question to mean: 'Do you have the ability to open the door for me?', not the 'hidden' prompt to actually do so. Somebody saying: 'Don't worry, it will pass', may be looked upon by the child with Asperger syndrome as a prophet who is able to literally look into the future. 'Give me your hand, I am just going to draw some blood', may provoke extreme panic, because the child understands the sentence to mean, 'Cut off your hand and give it to me.' It would be easy to misinterpret the child's reaction, believing it to be a sign that he was frightened of having blood drawn. The whole thing would then get completely out of hand by the nurse adding: 'No, don't worry, just give me your hand.' The child, in fact, had no problem with having blood drawn, because, like quite a number of children with autism spectrum disorder, he was not very sensitive to pain.

Pragmatic difficulties are paramount. Even in cases with marvellous expressive skills, difficulties carrying on a conversation can be major. Responding to 'open-ended' questions (such as 'How was your day?') may be almost impossible. They may respond by saying 'What exactly is it that you want to know?' Most will prefer concrete questions that have only one 'right' answer. They themselves may like to ask such concrete questions of other people, hoping always to get the right response. It is as though they had watched the communicative interactions of other people and concluded that first there is a question and then there is an answer and then there is another question and another answer etc. Because they may fail to understand the purpose of most people's questioning (i.e. the retrieval of new information about the other person's thoughts, feelings, intentions etc.), they perceive of the question–answer sequence more or less as a game, almost like 'Jeopardy'. It is not about learning new things, it is about finding out that the other person knows the right answer. Therefore, it is very common for people with Asperger syndrome to ask endless questions about things to which they themselves already know the answer.

People with Asperger syndrome have great difficulty using the social context as a basis for understanding the underlying message when people converse. They appear not to understand that one and the same sentence may have different meanings in different social contexts. They often have great difficulty understanding that different word stress and intonation ('prosody') can change the meaning of what it is that other people want to convey.

Many individuals with Asperger syndrome speak in slightly muted, muffled or mumbling ways, particularly when it is important that they express themselves in a clear way. These same people may then overarticulate when they use social clichés. Some stumble over the words and may even have so-called 'cluttering' speech. The majority have a 'flat prosody', a monotonous voice, even though there may be great variation in the degree of monotony. Pitch is often unusual, and voice control unadjusted to the social situation. Many speak too loud, low, fast or slow. There appears to be a deficiency in the auditory feedback system such that the person with Asperger syndrome may not actually hear that they are speaking too loud or too low.

Recent research has put emphasis on the issue of slowness in Asperger syndrome. Many people with Asperger syndrome are able to perform all sorts of laboratory tests aimed to reflect typical areas of everyday life impairments in the syndrome. However, they perform these tests very slowly, and may take twice or three times as long as other people to arrive at the correct solution. This slowness is sometimes very clearly mirrored in the way they speak or listen to other people. Only if you talk extremely slowly do they appear to be able to really listen to what you say. They themselves may then 'do socially better' if they respond very slowly. However, in ordinary social situations, conversations run at a high speed. The conversation may be filled with empty lacunas when the person with Asperger syndrome is attempting to process and understand what was said seconds ago. Perhaps this is one of the major reasons why people with Asperger syndrome have such enormous problems in real life settings even with the kind of social understanding that they manage relatively well in the laboratory.

In conversation with other people, the child with Asperger syndrome often demonstrates his inability to 'take in' the social situation and decide who is next in line in a conversation including more than two people. Utterances are pronounced without the slightest concern that some of the people involved in the conversation have no idea what is the actual topic. A number of 'in medias res' situations occur which, in intellectual and 'tolerant' settings may be interpreted as 'absurd' in a positive sense, but, which in other situations will almost invariably lead to major misunderstanding. Many boys with Asperger syndrome talk in an old-fashioned way, over-formally, almost as if they were reading out of an advanced textbook. They can have great difficulty even accepting that spoken language usually is not as perfect as written language and may feel 'offended' by the clutter and 'baseness' of ordinary conversation.

Some children with Asperger syndrome find that they are helped by making notes of what other people say so that they can then reanalyse the conversation when they are on their own. They often remember things that they have read (often also much better than same-aged children), even things they read years ago. At the same time they may have great difficulty remembering other than single sentences – often cut free from their context – of what they heard in a conversation in which they themselves participated only minutes ago. They may be better at remembering what they hear other people conversing about so long as there is no requirement for themselves to be part of the social context or the conversation. Thus, they may be both good observers and 'listeners', providing that they are not expected to partake in an ongoing interaction.

A characteristic problem is that they will not change their own wording or add extra information if, in a conversation, the partner appears not to follow the meaning or misunderstands something. Instead, the same sentence will be delivered over and over again, in spite of the conversation partner's questions, such as 'I do not understand what it is you're saying; can you explain?' Even when such questions are not pronounced by the partner, the context should have made it clear that he/she *heard* what was being said (and that therefore repeating it was uncalled for), but did not *understand* the meaning (which would have called for alternative explanations).

Communication problems affecting non-verbal skills

Non-verbal communication problems are paramount in Asperger syndrome. Facial mimicry may be extremely poor, gestures stereotyped, and the gaze stern, fixated, staring or wide-open. Some are said to have 'poker faces'. Many have problems judging appropriate physical distance when communicating with other people. They will come up too close or stand too far away from the person they wish to address or communicate with in other ways. The school-age child with Asperger syndrome may stand so close to the other person, that he/she may feel intimidated. The child may stare at the other person's mouth rather than his eyes and gestures and overall 'body language'. In another situation he may stand far away and even have his whole upper body turned away, so that it would be almost impossible for the person being addressed to know that he/she is expected to respond.

Asperger himself put considerable diagnostic weight on the intense, staring, penetrating gaze shown by many people with Asperger syndrome. From having being 'empty', 'dreamy', 'wide open', 'perplexed' or 'staring' in the early years in a majority of cases, a subgroup develops this type of very intense, fixating gaze around pre-adolescence. However, at least in my own experience, the wide-open gaze (with portions of the white showing above and below the iris) is at least as common.

There is often a naive, clumsy or merely restricted 'body language'. People with Asperger syndrome tend to lean in the wrong direction during conversation. They may place themselves behind the person they are talking to, start looking out the window at exactly the moment when contact around a certain theme is at its most intense, or get up and walk out in the middle of a conversation which was felt by the other person up until that point to have been meaningful and important. Very typical is the 'dead face', 'stone face' or depressed look, followed by the big smile, indeed sometimes laughter, as soon as the conversation comes to an end (as though from relief that there will be no further requirement for interaction). This latter symptom often remains one of the hallmarks of the syndrome in adult age.

Motor control problems

Motor coordination problems are typical of Asperger syndrome, and were highlighted in the early writings of Asperger himself. There is still little to support the notion that motor functions are 'damaged'. Nevertheless, people with Asperger syndrome can often be spotted because of their special, indeed sometimes very odd, motor performance. Their gait may be hypotonic, ungainly or stiff, often without accompanying arm swing.

Fine motor movements may be clumsy and ill coordinated, particularly in social settings. Some of those who appear to be the most clumsy can perform astonishingly well in activities for which the are highly motivated and well trained.

Gross motor performance, is, however, a big problem for the vast majority. This seems to be regardless of whether or not there is motivation. There may be problems with learning to ride a bicycle (many cannot do it at the age of 10 years), swim, catch a ball, or kick a ball in the right direction. Doing gross motor activities in a group can be even more troublesome. Many feel 'stupid' during physical education hours at school. Some may manage to kick a ball when on their own, but will be completely lost in the football (soccer) field.

Many of these with Asperger syndrome had some marked stereotypic movements in earlier childhood. Most of these will be gone by late childhood. However, there may still be some stereotypes, such as overstretched fingers close to the mouth, tightly held and shivering fists or minimal hand-flapping, that can all occur upon being excited. The excitement is often positive, but some stereotypies occur also when there is anxious waiting or worry. Stereotypies in Asperger syndrome are only rarely as marked as in classic variants of autism. School-age children with Asperger syndrome have often learned that other people regard stereotypies as something deviant and therefore actively try to 'hide them'.

Many children with Asperger syndrome develop tics around school age. Tics are not part of the syndrome but are so common and sometimes so difficult to differentiate from stereotypies and other motor control problems in Asperger syndrome, that they can cause considerable differential diagnostic problems.

Catatonia is another motor phenomenon that sometimes becomes a major problem in pre-adolescence. However, it is not part of the 'ordinary' motor control problems encountered in Asperger syndrome. The most common time period for its onset is in adolescence.

Summary of clinical picture

The symptoms described (poor social reciprocity, narrow interest pattern, ritualistic routines, speech and language peculiarities, non-verbal communication problems, and motor clumsiness) represent the clinical presentation of a typical boy aged 7–12 years with Asperger syndrome. They are also congruent with the diagnostic criteria for the condition outlined by Gillberg and Gillberg. Younger children, adolescents and adults, and girls, in particular, may show slightly different symptoms. In some cases, various kinds of comorbid problems may, at least for periods of time, overshadow the underlying Asperger problems and may contribute to the diagnosis being missed.

Symptoms in younger children are often somewhat more vague and it can be difficult, even for the experienced clinician, to decide which diagnosis within the autism spectrum – or, for that matter within the spectra of attention and tic disorders – is the most appropriate. There is sometimes a need to wait until the school year for 'classical' symptoms to emerge. This is one of the most important reasons why a diagnosis of Asperger syndrome is rarely made with confidence before school age.

Adolescents very often have additional problems (see below, chapter 5) and may also have 'learned' things about their problems (from reading or attending certain kinds of psychotherapy) that make it difficult to obtain a good history about primary symptoms and impairments. When problems have been misinterpreted for a long time and, for instance, been blamed only on school or parents, it can occasionally be extremely difficult to arrive at a reasonable assessment of the type and scope of the underlying problems.

Girls quite often do not have the typical patterns of special interests. However, some are so fixated on *social* routines or on other *people* that the fact that this fixation is really comparable to a boy's pursuit of another interest escapes you. Some girls are notorious 'refusers'. While boys may avoid demands by becoming irritated, chaotic, angry, or just sulking, girls quite often just 'disappear'. Without anybody later being able to explain just how she does it, the girl manages to avoid making a choice or complying with a demand. Other girls may avoid making choices by following in the footsteps of another, 'stronger' girl, and becoming their 'slave'. The language of some of the girls with Asperger syndrome whom I have met over the years has been less formal, less 'pedantic' than the language of similarly aged boys. At present, however, there is no good empirical data to suggest that girls with autism spectrum disorders generally differ from boys with similar conditions specifically in respect of language.

Bullying can lead to autism spectrum problems being missed

Children with Asperger syndrome often become the victims of bullying. In such cases it may take a very long time for an appropriate diagnosis to be established. From about age 10 years, many children with Asperger syndrome (at least one third) become depressed, sometimes in connection with bullying, sometimes not. Depression can also cloud the clinical picture and delay diagnosis of Asperger syndrome. A small proportion of those with Asperger syndrome commits severe antisocial acts (break-in and entry, fire-setting or violent crimes). They are often taken into the care of social authorities, and diagnosis of the basic impairments may be delayed for years, sometimes, probably, forever.

Autistic-withdrawn, active-odd, and passive-friendly subtypes of autism spectrum disorders

There are probably at least three major 'types' of presentation in Asperger syndrome: the withdrawn-autistic, active-odd and passive-friendly. These three 'variants' were first described by Wing (1989) in adults with autism, but it now seems clear that they also 'exist' in young children with Asperger syndrome. The descriptions are rough but excellent in that they each catch the 'gist' of the particular subtype already 'in the title'.

Emotions in Asperger syndrome

It needs to be emphasised that people with autism spectrum conditions are not unfeeling. Over the years, this has been one of the most widespread myths about autism. The reduced capacity for social interaction has led some experts to believe that underlying this is emotional coldness, and this belief has then been widely publicised. In the vast majority of cases, individuals with Asperger syndrome have strong feelings. Their problems lie in their failure to express or unusual ways of showing these emotions. Many with autism spectrum conditions are actually very good at 'picking up' feeling states. It is as though they have emotional antennae. However, they usually do not make appropriate sense of these perceptions and may very well misinterpret their 'intuitions'.

People with Asperger syndrome often behave in a chaotic fashion and seem to panic when subjected to mild or moderate stress or to specific perceptual stimuli for which they have poor tolerance. This is quite often mistaken as a typical panic attack and considered to reflect 'anxiety'. In a sense there is 'panic' and 'anxiety' but both will typically disappear almost instantly if stresses or the unwanted stimuli are removed.

Concluding remarks

Children with Asperger syndrome differ enormously in terms of social and academic handicap. The difference is often most marked in the early years and then tends to become less in a majority of cases. There are those who are suspected of suffering from autistic disorder in the first years of life, and some even receive that diagnosis – of autism or autism spectrum disorder – early on. Others are assessed for ADHD/DAMP or Tourette syndrome, and, in quite a number of cases, one, or more, of these diagnoses may be established. However, it seems that in a majority, while there has usually been some concern about social, language or behavioural development, no major psychiatric, personality or developmental disorder is suspected until into the child's school years. It is then that the classic picture that Asperger described emerges in a majority of cases. However, some, whose parents and teachers adopt a supportive 'personal assistance' strategy, may not 'decompensate' until late adolescence/early adult life, when they are left on their own to cope with the stresses of everyday life. Boys can usually be recognised and diagnosed in this age group, but many girls go unrecognised throughout this period. Comorbid problems, such as depression and anti-social acts, may obscure the clinical picture, so that a correct diagnosis may be missed for years. Otherwise it should be possible to detect and diagnose the vast majority of all clinically impaired children with Asperger syndrome during the early school years.

5

Symptoms in adolescence

It may be very difficult to recognise and diagnose Asperger syndrome during adolescence. This stems, in part, from the considerable comorbidity problems encountered in this age group. However, to some extent, it is also due to the fact that many adolescents with Asperger syndrome, just like other adolescents, want to be 'normal' and not to have any kind of functional impairments. Thus, any suggestion that their 'problems' might be 'symptoms' that are actually parts of a known 'syndrome' may be stubbornly rejected.

It is not uncommon for teenagers with Asperger syndrome to have major problems in the activities of daily life, such as personal hygiene, dressing, school work, eating and sleeping. Mild-moderate feelings of depression and irritability are common, as are various kinds of feelings of identity crisis. Drug abuse, and, albeit rarely, other types of antisocial activities, can occur, and can contribute to delaying the appropriate diagnosis of Asperger syndrome.

At least half of all teenagers with Asperger syndrome whom I have met do not manage personal hygiene in a satisfactory way. They may refuse to wash their hair or to take a shower, complain that the water 'feels strange when it comes in contact with the body', that soap and shampoo smell too strong or simply 'wrong', and object to washing private parts because it feels 'odd', 'stings' or 'is forbidden'. Other family members have sometimes come to accept that he/she will only agree to take a shower, or have a bath or a hair-wash once every two weeks or even more rarely. The hated procedure then takes place under great calamity, and it is not uncommon for all the other members of the family to have to be involved in one way or another. Much to the surprise of everyone, a teenager who has refused to cooperate in this manner for years, may suddenly accept the advice given by a doctor, teacher or psychologist to change to a new routine, namely taking a shower *every day*. The individual with Asperger syndrome is usually dependent on routines and often obsessive about them. A routine involving *daily* washing may be much easier to accept than one that involves having to choose between washing and no washing. There are sometimes such great problems with bodily hygiene, including a bad smell, that measures need to be taken to alleviate these before it is possible to get any further regarding diagnosis and work-up. However, the mere existence of major hygiene problems in a teenager should prompt suspicion that there might be an underlying autism spectrum disorder.

Dental hygiene can also be a major problem. Some children with Asperger syndrome have such severe perceptual problems relating to the gums and mucous membranes of the mouth that tooth brushing is experienced almost as though the nerve ends themselves were being brushed. For similar reasons it may be impossible to get them to the dentist. The perceptual problems in the oral cavity are usually reduced considerably by adolescence, but the fixated idea that tooth brushing is terrible and impossible remains. However, contrary to popular belief, there are few who refuse to go to the dentist because of other feared pain, pain that might frighten normally developing individuals from going to the dentist.

There are, perhaps I should say, of course, also those individuals with Asperger syndrome who are almost excessively perfectionist about their appearance and hygiene, and those for whom such matters are no problem whatsoever. A small number actually develop severely compulsive washing rituals, and may need specific help in alleviating these.

Hair and nail cutting may be major problem areas. The teenager may complain that 'it hurts', that he cannot cope with 'the sound of the scissors', or simply say that he 'has decided not to cut his hair anymore'. Some individuals have had these problems since early childhood but in many they become particularly problematic only in adolescence.

The teenager with Asperger syndrome may be orderly in the extreme when it comes to his desk drawer while at the same time allowing the clutter and chaos of the rest of his room to impede any activity. This is not exclusive to adolescents with autism spectrum disorders, but the contrast between the passionate pedantry reflected in the desk drawer and the filth and chaos in the 'big perspective' is often dramatic.

Some teenagers will wear the same clothes or shoes day in and day out for months, even years. They may throw tantrums if they discover that their clothes have been washed. After the washing, they complain that the clothes no longer 'feel right' or 'smell right'. Parents may have to wash, dry and iron the clothes during the night and then try to wrinkle them and keep them in the kitchen while frying something so that they will look and smell as though they had been used for a long time. Others are virtual snobs, and constantly demand new clothes. Some even change their clothes and shoes several times a day.

There are often major problems with school work. The teenager with Asperger syndrome sometimes does not realise the importance of good performance at school and feels that the teachers are to blame if they cannot get their pupils enthusiastic enough to do their best. There is, to an extent, perhaps some truth in this. Nonetheless, most teenagers realise that they themselves, not the teachers, will suffer most from not putting in a good effort at school. I have had patients who have told me that 'they have themselves to blame', meaning that the teachers are the only ones who have failed. It can be almost impossible to convince them of the need to devote more time and energy to school work. Considering the usually good rote memory skills, certain aspects of school work should be particularly easy for the individual with Asperger syndrome.

During the later school years, various kinds of group activities often hinder academic development in autism spectrum disorders. Many teenagers with Asperger syndrome find it impossible to work in a group, mainly because of the social demands and inability to adjust to common rules. However, sometimes they may take command of a group, perform the whole task by themselves and become appreciated by their classmates because nothing was required of them.

Bullying is sometimes the major problem. This may be open scapegoating or physical aggression, but sometimes it is a matter of silent exclusion. Bullying is probably a much under-rated phenomenon in Asperger syndrome. To some extent this may be attributable to the seeming lack of reaction on the part of some individuals with the condition. There are also those instances when age peers actively try to bully a teenager with Asperger syndrome, but he/she reacts so little or not at all that the perpetrators lose interest.

Asperger syndrome always needs to be considered in anyone who applies for psychiatric help in their teens. It is particularly important to be aware that underlying teenage depression, social phobia, OCD and eating disorder may well be an autism spectrum condition. Also, in cases primarily suspected of schizophrenia, perhaps because of a seeming regression in development, Asperger syndrome should be considered. It is not uncommon for high-functioning autism spectrum disorders to have *reported onset* around the time of adolescence when social demands and peer pressure increase, and family support is expected to decrease.

The individual with Asperger syndrome who seemed active and odd in childhood may well develop social phobia in adolescence. The awareness of being unusual, and, in so many ways, different from age peers, may lead to increasing feelings of social incompetence, and, hence, withdrawal.

Those who were passive as young children in my experience tend rather towards mild depression. They often do not actively withdraw, but because of their 'subdued' personality feel that their efforts at social interaction fail or are not 'appreciated' by other people.

The ones who seemed more withdrawn and 'autistic' in childhood often do not change style in adolescence. However, sometimes there is a seemingly abrupt onset of catatonic features. In retrospect one may find that there were mild catatonic symptoms long before adolescence, but these were not then handicapping and may therefore have been disregarded.

Girls and, more rarely, boys, with – often previously undiagnosed – Asperger syndrome may develop anorexia nervosa in adolescence. This, on more careful clinical analysis, is often an exaggeration of a long-standing problem with eating. Fixed ideas about 'appropriate foods' and various ritualistic phenomena have been present since early childhood but come to the forefront in adolescence. These – rather than the underlying autism spectrum problems – are then 'recognised' as a disorder that is well known among health officers working with adolescents, namely anorexia nervosa. It is important in such cases to diagnose the underlying autism spectrum problems, because interventions that are normally helpful in patients with eating disorders may be less than adequate in Asperger syndrome.

Concluding remarks

There are usually major associated and comorbid problems in Asperger syndrome in adolescence. Problems affecting the activities of daily life, such as personal hygiene and feeding, are commonplace. Depressed mood, victimisation, school problems in spite of good intelligence, and eating disorders are just some of the things that can contribute towards obscuring the nature of the underlying autism spectrum problems for a long time. Adolescence, in addition, is the age period when it is often least acceptable to the individual to even discuss the nature of the underlying diagnosis. This makes it a particularly difficult task to suspect, work up and diagnose Asperger syndrome in teenagers.

Associated psychiatric and social problems

There are many possible comorbid problems in Asperger syndrome. In fact, there is no other problem or diagnosis (except perhaps another disorder from the autism spectrum and severe mental retardation) that rules out a diagnosis of Asperger syndrome. Some of the most common and important comorbidities and associated problems will be described briefly here.

ADHD

In the vast majority of those with Asperger syndrome there are additional problems with attention deficits of various types. Such deficits, in turn, are often combined with motor coordination problems and other disorders of movement (including catatonic features). Sometimes, the attention deficits are of the extent and type encountered in ADHD and may be combined with overactivity and impulsivity. In other cases, it is more a question of exaggerated slowness and perfectionism leading to the individual not being sufficiently attentive to what goes on in the environment. The child – and adult for that matter – may quite simply be so absorbed by the task at hand that he/she may not notice, or does not care, that parents, teachers, psychologists or doctors are asking them to shift their attention to another task.

In one Swedish study, the great majority of all children meeting diagnostic criteria for Asperger syndrome also met criteria for ADHD with DCD (equals DAMP). Conversely, only a minority of all individuals meeting diagnostic criteria for DAMP show the full syndrome of Asperger's. This is accounted for by the relatively high prevalence of DAMP, and the much lower rate of Asperger syndrome in the general population.

A number of studies have been performed with the aim of analysing in more detail the attentional deficits encountered in ADHD, DAMP and Asperger syndrome. In spite of the fact that doctors, psychologists and teachers seem to agree that there may be differences across these groups both in the quantity and the quality of the attentional deficits, research so far has not been very successful in sorting out just what those differences might consist of at the neuropsychological level. Children with Asperger syndrome often – although by no means invariably – come across as more pedantic and slower than those with ADHD/DAMP who are often perceived as fast, impulsive and, even, sloppy.

Individuals with Asperger syndrome are often thought to be 'day-dreamers'. They appear to be not quite 'there', to be in their own world and to be thinking about something completely different. Attention to what goes on in the environment appears to be minimal. Oddly enough, he/she may suddenly demonstrate that all senses appear to have been 'on' all the time. Observations may have been made which were believed unthinkable given the degree of aloofness and withdrawal. It is as though the individual with Asperger syndrome were the sufferer of some kind of 'on/off-state' during which attention about what goes on in the environment is switched on only for brief periods of time, and it is during these seconds that astute observations are registered.

Tics and Tourette syndrome

Tics are extremely common in Asperger syndrome. In a Swedish population study, 80% of those with definite Asperger syndrome and 60% of those with definite or suspected Asperger syndrome had tics of one kind or another. At least 1 in 10, possibly 1 in 5 of all schoolchildren with Asperger syndrome have full-blown Tourette syndrome also. This is an extremely high rate compared to its prevalence in the general population.

The rate of Asperger syndrome in those having Tourette syndrome is also much higher than in the general population. About 1 in 20 with Tourette syndrome have typical Asperger syndrome, and another 3 in 20 have another kind of high-functioning autism spectrum disorder (Kadesjö and Gillberg 2000).

Affective disorders

Depression

Depression is probably the most common erroneous diagnosis in Asperger syndrome. Many people with Asperger syndrome look depressed with their reduced range of facial expression, clumsy and, perhaps, sluggish, motor movements, and seemingly disinterested way of 'conversing' about ordinary everyday matters. A label of 'depression' in such cases may be a total misnomer. The person with Asperger syndrome may be completely contented, at least with him/herself. He/she may feel that other people are a nuisance with all their demands for various types of interaction; if only people would leave them alone, things would be so much better.

At the same time, it is important to point out that many individuals with Asperger syndrome do develop depression. This is usually of the so-called reactive type. In such cases, depressive symptoms gradually worsen as the person becomes increasingly aware of being an outsider, having some functional impairments and being 'handicapped'. This is probably most pronounced in late pre-adolescence, middle teenage and early adult life. Protracted depressive episodes may occur and linger for more than a year until proper treatment – individual talks sometimes combined with antidepressive medication – is commenced.

A smaller group of all those with Asperger syndrome have episodes of endogenous depression, i.e. time-limited periods of depressed mood, sleep disturbance, anxiety in the early morning, and a variety of somatic complaints. These episodes do not show a clear temporal relationship with environmental triggering factors or with increasing insight into the nature of the functional impairments underlying Asperger syndrome. Rarely, such episodes can occur during the natural course of manic–depressive illness (see below).

Dysthymia

Dysthymia is listed as a special variant of depression in several diagnostic manuals. The differentiating features *vis-à-vis* depression (or rather depressive episodes) is that the depressed mood is more or less a chronic condition, and that the symptoms of depression are not severe enough to warrant a diagnosis of 'depressive episode'. Some individuals with Asperger syndrome not only appear to be chronically 'down', but actually are constantly in a low mood or outright depressed. They may be known as 'pessimists' and be more or less obsessed with various death themes. Others are irritable, tend to sulk and may be perceived as 'bitter'. Others still may be very tearful and whining.

Manic–depressive disorder

A depressive episode is sometimes a part of a depressive illness (also referred to as bipolar disorder). In this condition, the affected individual has episodes of mania (or hypomania) as well as of depression. Severe depressive illness is relatively rare in the general population, affecting about 1 in a 100 individuals. Manic episodes rarely occur in isolation, without there ever being clear periods of depression.

Even though no systematic study specifically looking at the rate of depressive disorder in Asperger syndrome has been published to date, clinical experience suggests that it is over-represented. Milder episodes of hypomania appear to be very common in Asperger syndrome and may show as increased activity or restlessness, increased talkativeness, more pronounced difficulties concentrating, decreased need for sleep, over-familiarity or unexpected sociability, or as overspending or other types of reckless or irresponsible behaviours. In frank mania such problems become much more severe. In addition there are usually feelings of inflated self-esteem or grandiosity and sexual activity may be much increased.

Some studies indicate that there may be a genetic link between high-functioning autism spectrum disorder (including Asperger syndrome) and depressive illness.

Atypical manic episodes

Episodes of increased activity coupled with marked irritability appear to be common in Asperger syndrome. The individual may not meet criteria for mania or hypomania, but there is nevertheless a clear change in behaviour which usually seems unrelated to external events.

Suicidal thoughts and acts

Suicidal thoughts are very common in Asperger syndrome. They appear to be particularly frequent in adolescence and early adult life, but can occur already at age 7 years. Some individuals with Asperger syndrome are so preoccupied with thoughts about death from an early age, that they begin to talk about 'suicide' in ways that, naturally, frighten their parents. It is of some interest that Hans Asperger, who noted this preoccupation with death in his patients, was himself fascinated by death. The only theme, other than autistic psychopathy and *Heilpädagogik* that he ever really wrote anything on was death.

A 10-year-old with Asperger syndrome may well say aloud that he is so bored with life he might just as well kill himself. Those who hear such words from a young boy usually become very upset, and some may seek psychiatric help for their child specifically because of such an utterance. Even though I know dozens of individuals with Asperger syndrome who started talking about death wishes, suicide and the like already long before adolescence, I have never yet seen one who actually did try to commit suicide at such a young age.

However, from about the time of puberty, suicidal acts become quite frequent. Some who commit such acts and who do not succeed have told me afterwards that they really wanted to die when they took the pills or tried to hang themselves, but the next day (and several weeks later) they felt very different about it. Some have tried to kill themselves because a schoolmate shouted 'Go kill yourself!' in anger. Bullying and a feeling of not being able to cope with all the social demands that life makes from around the time of puberty appear to be the most common triggers of suicide attempts, at least in this age group.

It is not uncommon for boys with Asperger syndrome to use violent methods if they try to commit suicide (hanging, shooting, poison, jumping from a bridge or in front of a train).

I have found that it can be very helpful to say to the person with Asperger syndrome: 'I do not think it is a good idea for you to try to kill yourself. For one thing, if you do not succeed, you may well end up brain damaged, and that would not be good for you.' I know at least a handful of individuals with Asperger syndrome who never repeated a suicide attempt after a psychiatrist told them something along those lines.

Alcohol and other drug abuse

It is also quite common for people with Asperger syndrome to start drinking a lot of alcohol towards the end of adolescence. This may sometimes be in response to peer pressure. In other instances, the person with Asperger syndrome may have noted that getting drunk takes him/her 'away' from the social demands of the situation. A Swedish and a British study both suggest that the rate of alcohol abuse may be extremely high in Asperger syndrome. When people with Asperger syndrome abuse alcohol it is often according to a pattern which sets them apart from others who abuse. They seem to decide on the exact quantity that they aim to drink every day, and then make it a 'golden rule' to stick to that routine.

In my clinical practice I have also seen a number of individuals who have experimented with a number of drugs other than alcohol. However, as yet, I have little idea of the scope of this problem in the general population of people with Asperger syndrome. Smoking is also quite common, but again, there is no evidence that it is more or less common than in the general population.

Interestingly, as with suicide acts, it may be possible to get some alcohol abusing people with Asperger syndrome to quit drinking merely by telling them that they should do so because it is not good for them to drink so much.

Eating disorders

Abnormal eating behaviours are almost the rule in Asperger syndrome (see chapter 4). Even though there are few formal studies documenting a relationship between autism spectrum disorders and disturbed/unusual eating behaviours, there is ample clinical evidence that such an association exists. Many people with autism spectrum disorders refuse to eat other than a very small number of dishes (such as French fries from MacDonald's, pickled herring, uncooked pasta or boiled rice). Some say they feel nauseated by certain food and insist on eating only things that 'do not smell'. Many start to 'sort' their food on the plate very early in life in a fashion very similar to that encountered in anorexia nervosa. There are those who refuse almost to drink (including drinking water) and say they never feel thirsty.

Some parents have told me that the most difficult symptom their child with Asperger syndrome had was to do with abnormal eating behaviour.

According to several Swedish studies, young women with anorexia nervosa may have Asperger syndrome or another autism spectrum disorder at a much increased rate. According to at least one German study, some young men with Asperger syndrome gradually develop such abnormal eating behaviours and become so thin that a diagnosis of anorexia nervosa is considered. Bulimia nervosa, on the other hand, does not appear to be associated with autism spectrum disorders.

Confusion states

In moments of stress it is not uncommon for people with Asperger syndrome to react with panic, 'hysteria', primitive reactions, fear, rage or childish tantrums. Such reactions may border on, and indeed sometime develop into, confusion states, during which it is quite impossible to reason with the affected individual or even to establish any form of 'contact'. The person affected may actually lose all sense of self, time or location. He/she may run about wildly, scream, throw him/herself on the floor or slam or even smash doors. I have seen men and women with Asperger syndrome break mirrors, run their arms through windows, and I have heard about those who ran straight into a stream of traffic or out onto the motorway without seeming to see or hear anything. The stress that provokes these kinds of reactions may be perceived by other people as very mild, or even to be something that they would have thought of as very positive. It could be anything from the wrong phrase spoken by somebody with whom the Asperger person is having a discussion, to the wrong sound or the wrong smell, or a demand which the Asperger person finds overwhelming (but about which he does not inform the stunned people who cannot understand why a tantrum/hysteric reaction occurs).

Negativism

Saying 'no', sulking or just 'being bored' are all very common in Asperger syndrome. In this sense, 'negativism' is extremely common in the disorder. However, there are those who are much more extreme in their negative outlook on life. It is not really that they are typical pessimists, rather that they constantly complain about everything, about other people and all their faults (some of which they may have themselves but seem not to be aware of), and that they complain about being slighted, oppressed, misunderstood and maltreated (even when there is good evidence that other people have treated them very fairly).

Catatonia

One of the most common types of motor problems encountered in high-functioning autism spectrum disorders is the phenomenon referred to as catatonia. Catatonia is seen in its most severe variant in individuals who 'freeze' as they move through a room, and are halted in mid-action. They literally remain in a particular posture for minutes, sometimes even hours.

Some recent studies suggest that about 10–20% of all individuals with autism and IQs above 50 may have moderate to marked features of catatonia. The risk of developing catatonia appears to be greatest among those who have an early history of language delay and who belong in the passive subgroup of autism spectrum disorders (Wing and Shah 2000).

Schizophrenia

Schizophrenia is probably not overrepresented in Asperger syndrome. However, it is not uncommon for individuals with Asperger syndrome seeking adult psychiatric help to receive this diagnosis. Some patients in my practice have been 'misunderstood' upon arrival in a psychiatric emergency ward after having appeared 'psychotic' or 'confusional' in connection with some rather minor incident that they experienced as awfully stressful. The psychiatrist in one such case asked: 'Are you hearing voices?' whereupon the person with Asperger syndrome responded 'Yes'. He received a preliminary diagnosis of 'psychosis with auditory hallucinations' which was soon changed to 'schizophrenia?' Much later, the patient himself said that in the chaos of the emergency room (and of his own mind) he thought the doctor was asking whether he could hear the voices of the other people in the room.

The problem is that when adult psychiatrists are not aware of the typical impairments of Asperger syndrome, they tend to see the dramatic presenting symptoms (which are definitely, in some cases, in one sense 'psychotic') and want to classify them according to a well-established terminology known to them. Once a diagnosis of 'schizophrenia?' has been made, it can be very difficult to change it. Schizophrenia currently carries a lot of treatment connotations that do not pertain to Asperger syndrome. For instance, while neuroleptics are considered part of the basic treatment curriculum in schizophrenia it is not a common option for Asperger syndrome.

It is possible that quite a considerable proportion of individuals attending adult psychiatric services with diagnoses of schizophrenia, 'schizophrenia?', schizophreniform psychosis, or psychosis NOS actually have 'underlying' undiagnosed Asperger syndrome or another autism spectrum disorder.

Personality disorders

Personality disorders are often diagnosed in individuals who have had autism spectrum disorder since early childhood. Unlike in the case of schizophrenia, such diagnoses are not symptomatically inappropriate: the patients actually meet criteria for many of these disorders (perhaps particularly obsessive–compulsive, schizoid, narcissistic, paranoid, schizotypal, avoidant and borderline personality disorder). The question is whether it adds anything to the understanding of the person with Asperger syndrome to say that he/she *also* has this or that personality disorder.

Antisocial development

It is easy, at least superficially, to confuse 'psychopathy', 'a lack of feeling', 'emotional coldness' and 'inability to feel remorse' with some of the symptoms of Asperger syndrome. Many have wondered about Asperger's own use of the word psychopathy in his paper on 'autistic psychopathy'. It is important to remember that psychopathy in older literature was more or less synonymous with the current concept of personality disorder.

Different from the person with psychopathy, the individual with Asperger syndrome can feel remorse. However it may be hard to admit to having made a mistake, and the feeling of being in the wrong can have been strongly resisted and discussed at length, either 'internally' within the person him/herself or in interaction with other people. People with Asperger syndrome are often perceived of as 'know-alls', which is unusual for people with psychopathy, who instead manipulate their environment and may agree to anything in order to come out 'on top'. The person with Asperger syndrome is rarely able to premeditate his actions for his own best and may stubbornly defend a position that is socially impossible and designed to put its proponent at a disadvantage. People with Asperger syndrome are often at their best in a one-to-one relationship, while those with psychopathy tend to be more at ease in a group where they are in a position to manipulate others. The individual with Asperger syndrome can seem to be unperturbed by the suffering of those who are near to them, but may be deeply involved in ethical, moral and philosophical issues. At work or in politics, they may be fighting for a good cause, something that would be unlikely, if not unheard of, in psychopathy.

A person with psychopathy is often considered charming by other people. However, he may also be seen as frightening, dominating and manipulative. It is definitely uncommon for him to be perceived as odd, weird or original/strange. In the case of Asperger syndrome, these are usually the first words to come to mind when trying to describe characteristic features of a person affected. Some are best described as stand-offish, aloof and difficult to come into contact with. Others are better recognised as naive, lost/helpless and touching. None of these descriptors are particularly appropriate in the field of psychopathy.

In 'real' psychopathy there may very well be good formal empathy skills, at least if empathy is seen as the equivalent of mentalising ability or having a theory of mind. The problem in psychopathy is that this ability to actually understand the thoughts and feelings of other people is not used in an affectionate, compassionate way, but only to enhance one's own persona or for personal gains.

Occasionally, one does come across an individual with Asperger syndrome who really strikes one as ice-cold, remorseless and manipulative – although in the latter instance, the 'art' of the manipulation is clumsy, and almost comical. It could be someone who may have difficulty separating dreams, fantasy and reality, and who – without the ability to judge other people's feelings and beliefs better – tells endless lies or plays so many roles that he has difficulty keeping track of them. Or it might be someone, who, lacking in distance and reflection, 'backstabs' other people, without seeming to understand that those people may be in daily contact with those receiving the negative information.

Antisocial – in the psychiatric sense of the word, i.e. breaking social laws in ways which are considered 'criminal' – development is probably not much over-represented in autism spectrum disorders. However, some individuals with Asperger syndrome, in their pursuit of a specific interest or in the course of a particular ritual, may commit crimes. Conversely, among criminals convicted for violent crimes and in whom forensic psychiatric evaluation has been undertaken, the rate of autism spectrum disorders is increased. Bizarre violent acts are only rarely committed by people with autism spectrum disorders. One such example is the killing of innocent people in an institution by somebody with Asperger syndrome, who many years previously had felt bullied by completely different people but in the same institution. There is a need for forensic psychiatrists to keep abreast of new information emerging in this field.

People with Asperger syndrome are, of course, 'antisocial' in other ways; such behaviours are part and parcel of the clinical picture. However, in the vast majority of cases, there is often rigid adherence to rules, and any unlawful activity would be unthinkable. Physical violence is completely revolting to many. Thus, even though severe antisocial and criminal acts occur in a few cases, and Asperger syndrome may be over-represented among some groups of offenders, people with autism spectrum disorders generally are certainly not dangerous and do not pose 'a threat' to society!

Concluding remarks

A number of other psychiatric diagnoses and personality disorders need to be considered in relation to Asperger syndrome. ADHD, DCD and other motor control problems (including catatonia), affective disorders, drug abuse and eating disorders are all common co-morbid problems. Schizophrenia and personality disorders are often diagnosed in Asperger syndrome, either mistakenly or because the diagnostician was not aware of the more informative diagnosis of the developmental autism spectrum disorder.

Other problems

Children with Asperger syndrome are at increased risk of a number of other problems, including academic failure, hyperlexia, problems that may arise on the basis of the child's high intelligence, lack of appropriate stimulation and bullying. Handicapping motor incoordination problems and general clumsiness may lead to a negative attitude to physical education (and appearing 'in the nude' in front of other children), and ball games. Balance problems may lead to 'high anxiety'. Perceptual problems – including auditive, sensory and olfactory ('smell') problems – may lead to avoidance of noisy environments, failure to attend to clothes and personal hygiene, preoccupation with certain materials and clothes, and systematic avoidance of specific foods.

School and learning difficulties

Many children with Asperger syndrome manage school without major difficulties – at least if the school has some (considerable) tolerance for unusual and eccentric people.

Some people with Asperger syndrome have specific learning difficulties. A few of these have dyslexia. However, dyslexia is common in the general population – affecting a certain percentage of school-age children – and it seems unlikely that it is exceptionally common in Asperger syndrome. Dyscalculia (specific problems in mathematics), on the other hand, may well be overrepresented in Asperger syndrome. Having said this, it may be important to point out that some affected children and adults are outstanding mathematicians. Attention deficits are extremely common in high-functioning autism spectrum disorders (including Asperger syndrome), and this often leads to a lack of interest in many school subjects. Achievement in these subjects is consequently affected, and it is quite common for highly intelligent individuals with Asperger syndrome to be severely underachieving. Quite a number seem disproportionately unconcerned by their own poor results in various school subjects. This would be particularly likely to occur if teachers or parents do not point out to them the sometimes very negative consequences of school failure.

Hyperlexia is a relatively common phenomenon in Asperger syndrome. In hyperlexia, the individual has a reading capacity usually well above that of age peers, and test results for reading are much superior to those expected on the basis of tested IQ. However, in most cases, the hyperlexia is mechanical in that the child can read perfectly from a written text, particularly if he or she is requested to read aloud. There may be major difficulties with silent reading and reading comprehension. Nevertheless, a considerable minority of all those with Asperger syndrome have true hyperlexia in that their relative capacity in all aspects of reading (mechanical reading, spelling, memorising, comprehension) is superior.

Perceptual problems

Perceptual problems are commonplace in Asperger syndrome. In a sense, Asperger syndrome is *a disorder of unusual perceptions*. Sound, vision, smell, taste, touch, heat, cold, pain – all may be perceived in ways which would be considered 'abnormal', 'incomprehensible', 'crazy' or even 'psychotic' by other people.

Unusual reactions to sound – ranging from panic at specific 'noises' (considered unobtrusive or even inaudible by others) through repetitive clinging to a certain tonal sequence – are almost universal. The specific adherence to certain language and speech characteristics, including the odd insistence on unusual dialects shown by some individuals with the syndrome, may also be a reflection of the unusual auditory perception. The fascination with word sounds and pronunciation may also be reflective of the unusual auditory perceptual 'style' of people with Asperger syndrome.

Fixation on aspects of the visual environment is also often, albeit not universally, encountered in Asperger syndrome. This could be shown by the odd staring at people and things, the tilting of the head to obtain an 'unexpected' or 'interesting' angle, and the flickering with various kinds of light that is so common in all autism spectrum disorders (not just Asperger syndrome).

Unexpected reactions to smell are so common in Asperger syndrome that most people living with it are unaware of their impact. The perception that a person 'smells' may be the only reason a person with Asperger syndrome avoids another human being. Nobody else may be aware of this smell (which may even be perceived as a 'stench' by the person with Asperger syndrome). Since the individual with Asperger syndrome does not share with other people what he/she experiences, there is no way that other people can understand some negative behaviours towards or even active withdrawal from some individuals. Unusual olfactory perceptions may also explain why some individuals with Asperger syndrome avoid some rooms or specific settings. A piece of cheese, raw lamb chops or cigarette smoke may be so obnoxious to the person with Asperger syndrome (child or adult) that he/she may avoid anything that would mean coming close to the source of the smell. Certain individuals with Asperger syndrome have great difficulty coping with gentle touch, but may love rough and tumble games or firm hugging. Some have clearly decreased pain sensitivity, but may be perceived as fussy because they cannot stand the various procedures and interactions following on an event that other people may have deemed painful.

Sensitivity to heat and cold may be altered in any direction. It is quite common for people with Asperger syndrome and other autism spectrum disorders to be able to tolerate heat and cold at levels that would be completely unacceptable to most other people.

Many with Asperger syndrome are panic-stricken at the sight, feel or mere knowledge of a 'stain' on a garment. Some refuse to change clothes because they cannot tolerate the new smell or unaccustomed feel of the texture of those clothes. It is quite common for people with autism spectrum disorders – including Asperger syndrome – to insist on wearing exactly the same shirt or dress day in and day out. Again, there are those who demand constant changes of clothes. A few of these individuals have told me that it was their need to find the 'perfect' garment that might match all their various perceptual peculiarities: a shirt, trousers, underwear with exactly the right smoothness, right smell and right colour.

Motor control problems

The majority of those with Asperger syndrome have motor incoordination or motor 'fluency' problems of various kinds. According to Asperger's view, and included among the current diagnostic criteria according to at least one manual, motor clumsiness is an almost invariable feature of the syndrome (see chapters 4, 5 and 6, in particular).

Apart from these relatively subtle motor dysfunctions, which are commonly perceived by lay people to be little more than 'normal' fumbling, stumbling and overall clumsiness, particularly in social situations, there are also more pronounced problems in some individuals. Problems of balance, sometimes bordering on mild 'ataxia', are not uncommon and may lead to refusal to climb (or, more commonly, descend) stairs without clinging to a person or a banister. Some of these may be struck by 'high anxiety' when standing on a small chair at the age of 5–10 years. Reduced or increased muscle tone may cause problems of posture and may lead to gait being either 'floppy' or very 'stiff'. It is possible that Asperger syndrome and other autism spectrum disorders may be overrepresented in certain variants of cerebral palsy, but this remains to be shown in systematic empirical studies. Many experience the motor problems either as incapacitating or at least severe enough to make participation in physical education 'impossible'.

As mentioned earlier, tics and Tourette syndrome are common comorbid features of Asperger syndrome. The tics can sometimes be difficult to distinguish from motor stereotypies, and also from other abnormal movements. Several recent studies have suggested that the motor systems are impaired in a number of different ways in high-functioning autism and Asperger syndrome.

Some children with Asperger syndrome get very little physical training of any kind, partly as a consequence of these motor problems, but partly also, of course, because of rigid ideas and a general refusal to do 'new' things. Some of this behaviour may well be thought of as 'a cautious attitude'; 'will not involve themselves in potentially dangerous activities', or, just plain 'laziness'.

Prosopagnosia (failure to recognise faces)

There have been some published case reports on the co-occurrence of the phenomenon of prosopagnosia – failure to recognise faces – and Asperger syndrome. I have met quite a number of people with high-functioning autism who have a marked difficulty recognising other people's faces, both in real life and in photographs. Some of these individuals had excellent memories for details of those other people's faces and could report eye colour, nose shape, and cheek-bone structure in a way which most individuals would have difficulty doing. However, when it came to selecting the particular face from among a series of photographs of people they would not be able to identify him/her. One of my patients usually would pass me by if I met him in a crowd or walking alone along the street. I first thought he did not want to speak with me, or that he would not have other people know I knew him (outside the hospital area). However, on other occasions, when I came in my car, he would recognise me immediately and come up to say hello. It was not that he was fixated on cars and totally avoided people. He said he was not sure it was 'his' doctor until he saw the car. These problems, referred to as prosopagnosia, are sometimes quite similar to those observed in children with 'developmental visual agnosia', a condition in which children with normal visual acuity may have great difficulty orienting themselves in the visual environment.

To my knowledge, no larger-scale formal study has ever been performed to determine whether the rate of prosopagnosia is much raised in Asperger syndrome or not.

Concluding remarks

School problems are very common in Asperger syndrome, even in those who are highly intelligent. Many have great difficulty concentrating on and taking an interest in tasks considered important in the academic world, be it primary school or at the university level. A smaller group of individuals have specific learning problems. These may be particularly pronounced in the motor domains. Many have such great difficulty with motor coordination and other aspects of motor behaviour that they may need the skilled help of a physiotherapist. Perceptual problems are the rule, and they include overreaction to sound and abnormal reactions to smell, taste, heat, cold and touch. Some people with Asperger syndrome have specific problems recognising other people's faces and orientating themselves in a complex visual environment (even when they may have an excellent sense of 'locality'). For a rather small group of people with Asperger syndrome these associated problems of learning, motor control and perception are so pronounced as to comprise their greatest impairment.

Strengths

Virtually all children, adolescents and adults with Asperger syndrome have strengths and abilities that tend to contradict the impression of a person with 'impairment'. Some of these can actually be seen as aspects of the syndrome itself, whereas others are best understood in the context of each individual's unique personality. Many with the syndrome have good or even superior intelligence. However, it is not rare, even in such cases, to encounter cognitive difficulties that would not seem to fall into the social or behavioural domains. Special areas of expertise are quite common, which should come as no surprise given the symptom of narrow interest patterns that is part of Asperger syndrome. This interest may be so pervasive, and energy and motivation so strong as to lead to exceptional feats of work. Under such circumstances, productivity may occasionally be extreme. Rote memory is often very good, as is the ability to cover, and remember, large 'chunks' of written material. Some have eidetic ('photographic') memory. Perseverance and persistence may be pronounced personality characteristics that carry some very positive implications. Perfectionism is common, even though it is often limited to certain areas of functioning, and may well be coupled with a glaring lack of orderliness in other domains. I have had a clinical impression over the years that people with Asperger syndrome seem to age (physically) very slowly, at least in middle age: they very often look much younger than would be predicted by their chronological age.

General intelligence

Intelligence (Intelligence Quotient/IQ) is probably higher, on average, in a group of people with Asperger syndrome than in the population at large.

The difference may not be great, but is, nevertheless, remarkable given the many difficulties – social interaction problems, decreased ability to seek new knowledge through other people, the language and communication peculiarities, the lack of speed, motor control problems and attention deficits – that would contribute towards generally lower intelligence. This would argue in favour of 'basic IQ', i.e. the intelligence level that the individual would have been functioning at if they had not had the unusual developmental pattern/brain variation that causes Asperger syndrome, being much higher than in the general population. This would tally with the overrepresentation of highly intelligent or otherwise very 'gifted' parents commonly reported in Asperger syndrome. There has been speculation that high IQ might itself 'predispose' to Asperger syndrome in the offspring – and, there is definitely a problem of differential diagnosis when it comes to separating some cases of Asperger syndrome from merely extremely high intelligence. Asperger himself suggested that there might be such an association. It is of considerable interest that Kanner also felt that there might be just such a connection between parental high IQ and classic variants of autism. Regardless of this, high IQ is often the outstanding asset/strength in people with Asperger syndrome and must be acknowledged and taken advantage of. Instead of underscoring the social difficulties and putting all the money on developing social skills, one must emphasise the intellectual capacity and, in so doing, strengthen self-confidence. Even in cases with low abilities in non-verbal domains, some language skills may be extremely strong. Vocabulary, for instance, may be exceptionally good in spite of general IQ being in the low normal or slightly subnormal range.

Special skills ('savant' abilities)

The syndrome that Asperger described is characterised by narrow patterns of interest. Good, sometimes excellent, rote memory skills in combination with an obsessive–compulsive nature bordering on the ritualistic increase the likelihood that these narrow interests will lead to the amassing of knowledge and special abilities in certain areas. Such abilities, when extreme, and, particularly when unexpected given the overall level of intellectual functioning, are often referred to as 'savant' skills. This concept was first used in connection with people suffering from mental retardation who occasionally demonstrated such 'splinter' abilities; the term used originally was 'idiot savant'. It is very common for children and adults with Asperger syndrome to show exceptionally good knowledge in narrow, well-defined areas. Other individuals taking an interest in the same area would never dream of acquiring similar catalogue knowledge. Individuals with Asperger syndrome may show such knowledge even when their overall IQ is not exceptionally good.

Savant skills may occur in other conditions, and in normalcy. They are relatively much more common in autism spectrum disorders including Asperger syndrome. The term is now used for special talents at a very high level of functioning, much above that which would be expected on the basis of a person's IQ.

Rote memory and eidetic memory

About one-third of my patients with Asperger syndrome have exceptionally good rote memory skills. This may involve auditory as well as visual information. In the latter case, reference is often made to 'photographic memory' or 'eidetic memory'. Some individuals seem to remember, in a very concrete manner, everything they ever experienced, and may recapitulate, even 15 years after the event, a verbatim account of a conversation or a photographic description of a chain of development. The ability to differentiate between true and false memories may be particularly well developed in some individuals with Asperger syndrome. Some have exceptionally good orientation skills, but others, maybe because of a lack of central coherence or visuospatial problems (see chapter 11) show extreme difficulty orienting in new situations.

Persistence

Many with Asperger syndrome are impatient and tend to give up easily. Many others are extremely persistent. Others still combine impatience in some settings – usually those that are perceived as uninteresting or 'impossible' – with extreme tenacity and persistence in other situations – not least, of course, in areas of special narrow interests. All three groups have strengths. The impatient group may inspire other people to develop in directions that were previously believed to be impossible. The persistent group will return to a theme, persevere and carry out tasks that others would refuse to do because they were felt to be too 'dull'. In the group that oscillates between extremes, it is often difficult to keep track of changes and respond to them, but the fact that one individual may show both extremes may be a special strength.

Energy

Many with the syndrome are perceived by others as 'slow', 'lazy' or 'hypoactive'. A somewhat smaller group shows very high levels of energy, and may, particularly if there is a very strong interest and motivation is high, accomplish things that others would not feel up to. This may apply in respect of both intellectual and physical achievements. Feats of accomplishment may result if there is an interesting goal in sight.

Some of those with very high energy levels are perceived by other people as workaholics or even hypomanic or manic. Longer-term observation will mostly reveal that pathological overactivity is not present. However, in rare instances, manic hyperactivity does occur.

Perfectionism

Just as with persistence so it seems to be with perfectionism in Asperger syndrome. There is one group that appears to be careless, one (often exaggeratedly so) perfectionist, and one that fluctuates between extremes. The very perfectionist and 'mixed' groups can benefit greatly from their extreme demands in exactness, not least in technical or scientific matters.

Slow maturation – slow ageing?

My clinical impression over the years has been that people with Asperger syndrome mature slowly, and, in a parallel fashion, age slowly. In 'mature' age, many look much younger than their chronological age would suggest. Their hands and faces may be surprisingly smooth, as though 'unused', even in middle age. As young children these same individuals may have looked serious and 'overly adult'. As they grow older it is sometimes conspicuous how 'young', 'naive', 'childish' or even 'babyish' they may look. To some extent, the lack of non-verbal facial communication that is so often part and parcel of the syndrome, could contribute towards this impression. Unusual development of hormones or growth factors is, of course, an alternative explanation.

Concluding remarks

People with Asperger syndrome almost always have major strengths that may, wholly or partly, compensate for the major difficulties. Almost all the core features of the syndrome have 'positive' opposites. Good general IQ, perseverance, stubbornness and perfectionism are just a few of the strengths often shown by individuals with Asperger syndrome. It is always important to charter these strengths in connection with diagnosis and follow-up, so as to allow the best possible education, vocational training and overall development in each individual.

Background factors

It has not yet been definitely established what causes Asperger syndrome. A genetic contribution is clearly important in many cases. Some cases have been linked to damage or developmental abnormalities in the brain arising either in foetal life or in the first years after birth. It is possible that some instances of the syndrome are attributable to the combination of genetic and brain damaging events. Psychosocial factors in themselves appear to contribute little in terms of *causing* the syndrome, but may be very important from the point of view of outcome.

Genes

At least half of all children, adolescents and adults with Asperger syndrome have a close relative – parent or sibling – with similar, albeit not necessarily identical, problems. It has also been well established that some individuals with Asperger syndrome have children with similar, indeed sometimes almost identical, difficulties. However, it is far from clear how large a proportion of all those with Asperger syndrome are liable to have children with similar functional impairments.

Asperger syndrome is considered an autism spectrum disorder. That autism itself is a strongly genetic condition has been shown convincingly by several twin and family studies. Those studies have also demonstrated that in many cases it is not 'autism per se' that is inherited, but rather a broader range of autism spectrum problems ('autistic traits'). Family studies have shown clearly that autism and Asperger syndrome often occur within the same larger family tree. Full genome screen studies have been performed in autism. The results of these, combined with the data from twin and family studies, suggest that several different genes located on different chromosomes increase the susceptibility for autism and, when they act together, the full syndrome of autism results. There is some evidence that genes involved in the regulation of early hindbrain (brainstem) development may be important in autism spectrum disorders. Genes located on the X-chromosome, chromosome 15, and chromosome 7 have also been implicated in several studies. It seems likely that yet other gene locations are of importance for autism susceptibility.

It is not clear how genetic factors operate in Asperger syndrome. It is *possible* that a small proportion of cases may be due to autosomal recessive genes, i.e. both parents carry the same defective gene, although in their case that single defective gene has not led to disorder (because they both have another, non-defective copy of that gene). Yet other cases *may* be inheritable in an autosomal dominant fashion, i.e. be caused by one major gene contributed by one of the parents. Rare cases are caused by specific chromosomal disorders, such as the fragile X syndrome, XYY syndrome, XXY (Klinefelter) syndrome, translocation syndromes, or the CATCH-22 syndrome. However, the vast majority of familially transmitted cases of Asperger syndrome are probably due to so-called polygenic inheritance, i.e. several *susceptibility genes* act 'in concert' to produce the typical syndrome.

An increasing number of studies suggest that there are 'subclinical' variants of Asperger syndrome or high-functioning autism. Such cases, while demonstrating all the typical characteristics, have such mild symptoms or impairments that psychiatric, paediatric or psychological consultation may not be contemplated either by family members or the individuals themselves. In families containing children with classic Asperger syndrome there appear to be many more individuals with subtle, but similar personality traits that are strongly reminiscent of those encountered in the 'full-blown' syndrome. Perhaps if one child receives a 'large dose' of the susceptibility genes for Asperger syndrome (or for the 'broader autism phenotype'), he/she will present with the classical variant. Another child, in the same family, may receive a much smaller dose, or none of the required genes, and will show only a few or no symptoms of Asperger syndrome. In other families, both parents may have mild, sub-clinical traits of Asperger syndrome. It is possible that when their genes combine, they may do so in a way that leads to one, or more, of their children developing the typical, functionally impairing syndrome.

The subclinical variant of Asperger syndrome is often characterised by egocentricity, rigid thinking and inflexible behaviours, greed, perfectionism, 'unwanted-truth-telling' and, sometimes, a strong social interest/conscience but with little or no social talent. Major life issues, such as equality among men, justice, human rights, animal rights or political issues, may be pursued with great fervour, even when those same issues are being dealt with in everyday life in ways which others would perceive as clumsy and lacking in insight. Many are tellers of funny stories and anecdotes that are repeated endlessly in unvaried format. Some live alone or with their parents well into middle age. There was a time when such people were referred to as loners, eccentrics or just 'original people'. Some became isolated academics who would spend their lives delving into one or other area of their special interest. In modern societies, with ever-increasing demands on team-work, collaboration, and social interaction (at least in most areas), it is becoming more and more difficult for individuals with subclinical Asperger syndrome to 'remain subclinical' throughout the life-span. Social, including vocational, demands, social interaction in itself and 'stress' (not perceived by other people as particularly stressful) will eventually lead to such people developing major marital, family or work-related problems that will, sooner or later, require professional help. In such cases, with not much of 'a history', it may be particularly important to consider the possibility of Asperger syndrome.

Males are strongly overrepresented in the clinical variant of Asperger syndrome. Current models for understanding the genetics of autism spectrum disorders have not contributed a great deal to elucidating why this should be. Some of the salient features of Asperger syndrome could be construed as extreme exaggerations of what some people would refer to as 'the male psyche' (tendency to social isolation, formalism, subdued expressions of non-verbal communication, interest in only a few or narrow areas rather than a varied interest pattern). There is actually some, albeit limited, empirical evidence that this stereotype may not be a complete misrepresentation of realities. If, indeed, boys and men tend just a little bit towards the 'Asperger type personality', then a smaller gene dose or less severe brain damage would be needed to 'push' him 'over the edge' as compared with what would be required in the case of a female. This *could* account for some of the skewed gender ratio in Asperger syndrome. Related to this line of reasoning is the notion that girls/women with the core problems of Asperger syndrome may be missed in clinics where autism spectrum disorder is diagnosed. If females with the crucial characteristics show a slightly different 'phenotype' (roughly equivalent to 'symptomatic presentation') as compared with males, then the male prototype – which was certainly what Asperger described – connected with our conceptualisation of the syndrome would lead to underdiagnosis in girls and women. Several recent studies have argued that this may indeed be the case, and females may receive a host of other diagnoses, including obsessive–compulsive disorder/personality disorder, eating disorder or atypical depression, when, in fact, Asperger syndrome would have been a more appropriate (and more helpful) diagnosis.

Brain damage, brain dysfunction and brain variation

There are many different types of brain damage. The brain may be hit by brain damage universally or only in a highly specific and limited area. Asperger syndrome and other autism spectrum disorders can be caused by such brain damage. Asperger himself was convinced of the important role of damage to the developing nervous system in the causation theories he developed for autistic psychopathy. Some systematic studies exist that show a marked overrepresentation of such possible brain damaging factors occurring in foetal life, during birth or in the first few years of life in Asperger syndrome. It is often impossible to determine whether such suspected damage is the cause of the syndrome or perhaps a reflection of an underlying genetic factor that predisposed the foetus to unusual/abnormal development. The risk factors most often implicated in the literature on Asperger syndrome are deviant mode of delivery, 'artificial' delivery (such as by forceps), prematurity, postmaturity, low birth-weight, early membrane rupture, maternal alcohol abuse throughout pregnancy and so-called maternal toxaemia. As has already been mentioned, there is occasionally another medical disorder causing the brain problems that underlie the symptoms of Asperger syndrome (Marfan syndrome, XYY or CATCH-22 syndrome, to mention a few of the possible disorders).

Several researchers believe that genetic and brain-damaging factors may act in concert, the genes producing the substrate (precondition) for the disorder, which will only becoming clinically manifest if there is also added brain damage.

Brain damage can be structural and its consequences macroscopically visible upon inspection of the brain at autopsy or in connection with 'neuro-imaging' (CT or MRI scanning, for example). It is often microscopically discernible and objectively observable at histological examination of brain tissue at autopsy. However, in many instances, the brain dysfunction that follows brain damage is the only 'mirror' of the acquired or genetic lesion long after the actual 'event'. This can be demonstrated either neurophysiologically (for instance at EEG or ABR examination) or neurochemically (for instance, by analysing cerebrospinal fluid).

It is also possible that some of the 'symptoms' of Asperger syndrome should be interpreted as variation in brain function rather than as reflecting specific underlying damage, dysfunction or disorder. Such a view of the neurobiology of autism spectrum disorders is consistent with hypotheses that link Asperger syndrome to personality disorder and to the 'continuum of normality' typical of so many other human functions and 'traits'. Thus, it is possible that some of the hallmarks of Asperger syndrome should be seen rather as extreme variations of the normal distribution of social and behavioural functioning, not so much as a pattern signifying pathology in the more narrow sense of the word.

Where in the brain is Asperger syndrome?

Results from a considerable number of neuropsychological and neurophysiological studies indicate that many of the basic impairments in Asperger syndrome may be attributable to unusual or aberrant functioning in the frontal lobes – or in neighbouring areas in the frontal and temporal lobes. A reduction of so-called executive functions and of mentalising abilities (see chapter 11) is probably originally very often due, completely or partially, to deficient capacity in these areas of the brain. Indirect support for dysfunction of 'more primitive' areas of the brain – including the brainstem and the cerebellum – has also been contributed from the study of high-functioning individuals with autism.

In a joint London–Gothenburg study (Happé et al. 1996) we identified an area in the left frontal lobe (Brodmann area 8/9) which did not function in a 'normal' fashion in Asperger syndrome. Young men with Asperger syndrome were compared with normally functioning men on their ability to solve mentalising tasks (tasks that require empathy and the ability to see another's cognitive/emotional perspective) while undergoing an imaging study of brain activity (so called PET scanning). Normally functioning men activated Brodmann area 8/9 while solving the task, whereas the men with Asperger syndrome activated a different (neighbouring) area. The results could be taken to indicate that the reduced capacity for mentalising observed clinically in individuals with Asperger syndrome is closely related to deficient function in Brodmann area 8/9 in the left frontal lobe.

In another study using PET scanning and MRI, both individuals with 'high-functioning autism' and same-aged people with 'Asperger syndrome' showed reduced metabolism (and reduced volume) of portions of the gyrus cinguli of the limbic system, specifically Brodmann's area 24, compared to gender- and age-matched healthy volunteers (Ring et al. 1999).

There have also been studies of functional magnetic resonance imaging (fMRI) suggesting that individuals with Asperger syndrome do not activate the same brain areas as 'normal controls' when analysing facial emotions, and that they may use 'non-facial strategies' when studying human faces (Critchley et al. 2000).

Findings from other studies, such as the careful analysis of children undergoing work-up for epilepsy surgery, imply that the symptoms of Asperger syndrome may also result from lesions in the right frontal lobe (Taylor et al. 1999). Neuropsychological studies of individuals with so-called non-verbal learning difficulties (chapter 2) indicate that there is considerable overlap between this type of dysfunction and the clinical syndrome that Asperger described. Non-verbal learning difficulties are believed to be caused by dysfunction or damage to neural circuits in the right cerebral hemisphere.

One theory proposes that Asperger syndrome is caused by unilateral dysfunction of particular brain areas that are interconnected by the corpus callosum (the large brain structure that crosses the midline of the brain). Whenever there is dysfunction or damage on one side early in development, the corresponding site on the other side will 'try to take over' the function that was intended to have been developed by the abnormal area. Thus, even if mentalising skills were 'primarily' the 'task' of left frontal lobe areas and certain other communication skills the task of the right frontal lobe, dysfunction on any one side would reduce the capacity available for compensation by the other side. This would result in impairment of mentalising and other communication skills regardless of the side of the brain being affected by damage or dysfunction. However, impairment would not be extreme such as in the case of classic autism, which, under this model, would require bilateral brain abnormality.

It is early days yet in the field of Asperger syndrome brain research. All that has been achieved so far is the very small opening of a window onto understanding the basic brain mechanisms that underlie the complex web of symptoms encountered even in the most classic cases. The next 10 years will almost without doubt provide us with a much better brain conceptualisation of the syndrome.

Psychosocial factors

There is no evidence that Asperger syndrome can be caused by psychological or social factors. This is not to say that social circumstances cannot ever lead to biological hazards that can lead to the typical impairments seen in Asperger syndrome. For instance, it is clear that alcoholism in a mother can sometimes develop under conditions of severe psychosocial stress (even though maternal alcoholism may not be related to such stress at all). Alcohol can lead to foetal brain damage that may lead on to the symptoms of an autism spectrum disorder. However, the vast majority of children with Asperger syndrome grow up under conditions that are no different from those of 'normally functioning' children.

As with any chronic impairment or disease, social and psychological factors play a major role for the individual and his/her ability to lead a life without major handicap. There is emerging evidence that early diagnosis, information, psychological support and educational interventions can reduce suffering and degree of handicap in the longer term, both for the individual affected and his/her family. This, to a considerable degree, is the effect of changed attitudes and better understanding among the closest members of the social network. It has been mentioned several times already that individuals with Asperger syndrome may react with severe psychiatric breakdown under conditions of even mild stress. It goes almost without saying that in such circumstances, many psychological problems should be seen as 'secondary' and that they would be potentially preventable through changes in the attitudes of people living or working with those affected by Asperger syndrome. One study in our centre showed that families, teachers and peers who 'know' what it is all about, are much more positive in their reactions than those who do not have a name for the problems. They make much more appropriate demands and have more realistic expectations. This means that they can take the pressure off in some areas while having a more positive – and demanding – attitude in other fields. To some people this would seem to be self-evident. Unfortunately, there are still those who claim that diagnosing a problem is like 'branding the child'. However, failing to make a diagnosis of an autism spectrum disorder is much like, or even worse than, failing to make an appropriate diagnosis of a visual problem or a hearing deficit.

It is likely, although not yet shown in empirical study, that Asperger syndrome can remain a 'subclinical' problem or develop from a severe clinical condition into a subclinical one, if the psychosocial milieu takes into account the strengths, difficulties and basic personality of the affected individual.

Nevertheless, it has to be said that few conditions appear to be more difficult to change radically by changes in the environment. More than 25 years of experience has shown me this aspect of autism spectrum disorders to be perhaps more striking than any other. Meeting the person with Asperger syndrome at age 30 years and going through his current situation and comparing the findings with those of the notes of the medical records entered 23 years earlier, can be an almost unbelievable experience. Everything is the same, nothing has really changed, all the early problems are still there. Symptoms and outward presentation may, indeed will, have changed, but they still fall into the basic groups of symptoms described in chapter 4.

There may be psychosocial problems stemming from having a father or mother – or brother or sister – with the disorder or other symptom constellations in the autism spectrum. These will have to be dealt with in their own right and not mixed up with 'causation theories'. The reverse may also be true: having a close relative with an autism spectrum disorder may be very helpful in that basic understanding of the problems associated with it may be better developed under such conditions. Asperger described cases in which an affected mother or father was clearly the best support the child with 'autistic psychopathy' could have wished for. I have seen many such cases. Therefore, there can be no one view as to the implications, positive or negative, of having a close relative with the same, or similar, disorder. Every case has to be reviewed without prejudice.

Bullying at school, in the playground or in a group of age peers, can be a terrible psychosocial problem. It needs to be addressed immediately. It can often be prevented by early diagnosis and by informing people in the immediate environment. Children without Asperger syndrome sometimes do not tell their families that they are the victims of bullying; in Asperger syndrome one should definitely not expect the child to share information of this kind on his own initiative. One has to be aware of the very real possibility of bullying and ask appropriate and concrete questions. Only then can bullying be detected early in the process and terrible consequences avoided.

Perhaps I should also say that some individuals with Asperger syndrome are not perceived by their age peers as candidates for bullying. Instead, they may be thought of as 'detached', 'superior' or 'untouchable', even 'leaders', who would never be victimised. As previously mentioned, others may be exposed to bullying which may soon subside because the individual with Asperger syndrome does not react in the expected fashion.

Gender differences

There are possibly some differences in the clinical presentation of Asperger syndrome depending on gender. This has not yet been properly documented by large-scale epidemiological studies. In my experience, girls with Asperger syndrome are sometimes less aggressive, less prone to hyper-activity and not so fixated on specific narrow interests. They tend to be more interested in 'social' toys, such as dolls, whereas boys often demon-strate a stronger interest for hard objects, water, sand and mechanical things.

It is quite possible that all of these differences are to do with similar differentiating features across the genders in the general population. Never-theless, they may be important in that the male prototype for autism spectrum disorders is the one that has been promulgated almost exclusively over the last 50 years or so. Those few girls who have been diagnosed with autism in the past have usually been severely affected, often with major signs of brain damage. This could be because a large proportion of all girls with autism spectrum disorders – specifically those that are higher functioning – may have been undetected in these studies, conveying the false message that when girls have autism they are more severely handicapped.

Concluding remarks

What causes Asperger syndrome is not known but genetic factors and/or brain damaging events are believed to be the determinants of the disorder. There is no evidence that psychological or social factors themselves can cause the typical symptom constellation encountered in Asperger syndrome. This does not mean that psychosocial factors are unimportant. Indeed, they are crucial for the understanding of how to help individuals and families affected. It is possible that unilateral aberrant frontal lobe function is vitally important for human empathy skills, and that people with Asperger syndrome have empathy problems because of specific impairment of such brain function. The evidence is currently equivocal as to which brain hemisphere is most likely to be impaired in Asperger syndrome.

Cognitive neuropsychology

Cognitive psychology and neuropsychology have contributed important clues to the 'basic mechanisms' underlying autism spectrum disorders, including Asperger syndrome.

Several cognitive domains have been shown to be impaired or to function differently in autism spectrum disorders. Some of these domains represent overlapping constructs, and it is quite common in research to favour or focus on one of these rather than on all at the same time. This has led to the formulation of a number of interesting hypotheses regarding the 'true nature' of autism spectrum disorders. It may need to be stressed that no one of the various psychological functional impairments that will be described in this chapter excludes the coexistence of one or more of the others.

At least four areas of cognitive/neuropsychological functions appear to be impaired or atypical in autism spectrum disorders. These are (i) mentalising ('theory of mind'/'empathy') abilities; (ii) executive functions; (iii) drive for central coherence; and (iv) procedural learning. It is likely, although by no means yet certain, that all these areas are affected by impairment or atypical functioning early in the lives of those with Asperger syndrome. Later, there may be measurable dysfunction only in one, two or three of these areas, although the clinical impression may still be one of handicap in all four domains.

Mentalising, theory of mind and empathy

The ability to imagine other people's thoughts and feelings, indeed the ability even to attribute mental states to other people, is limited in autism. Mentalising abilities are severely impaired in all young children with classic autism. According to laboratory tests it is probably lacking altogether in the majority during the preschool years. Some of the most profoundly handicapped individuals with autism may be lacking mentalising skills throughout life. 'Typically developing' children demonstrate skills that probably reflect emerging, even good, mentalising skills in the first two years of life. For instance, they try through looking at other people to direct their gaze to objects or events that they have themselves observed. Also, they come to other people for comfort, help and information very early in life. Such behaviours are usually not seen at all in preschoolchildren with classic autism. Mentalising ability has also been referred to as 'theory of mind skills' by cognitive psychologists, and 'empathy' by child psychiatrists. Mentalising skills may be required in order to interpret the world and what goes on in it in abstract rather than concrete terms only. Given that, without a theory of mind, it would be impossible to attribute mental states to people, their actions would have to be interpreted in strictly behavioural terms. The actions of other people would be taken 'at face value' without an understanding of the underlying intentions, wishes, hopes or feelings. 'Common sense' skills would be deficient, unless specifically taught or rigorously 'trained'.

Mentalising is much less markedly impaired in laboratory tests of school-age children, adolescents and adults with Asperger syndrome, even in cases when the clinical impression would have suggested severe handicap in this field. However, although in the laboratory setting they may finally arrive at a 'correct conclusion', they often do so in laborious, oblique, unusual or tortuous ways. Mentalising ability can be conceived of as synonymous with empathy skills. Poor ability to mentalise would invariably infer deficient ability to take the perspective of others and hence poor ability to put oneself in another person's place. This is exactly the ability that is required for 'empathy'.

Clinical experience suggests that young children who later conform to the gestalt of Asperger syndrome lack mentalising ability in the first few years of life. When the ability finally emerges, it is delayed in its further development. Even when, in adolescence or adult age, formal mentalising tests are passed – with or without obvious peculiarities in the problem-solving style – mentalising skills are 'slow', 'sluggish', 'indirect', 'intellectual rather than intuitive' or simply not automatised. The individual with Asperger syndrome does not have the appropriate mentalising skills at the stage of development (say around age 2–5 years) when children (with well-developed skills in the field) are expected to interact reciprocally with age peers and train themselves in social interaction. This leads to an unusual quality of interaction and communication, one which may be felt by other people to be 'unnatural', 'stiff', 'formal', 'stilted' or 'rigid'. In direct contact with other people, the person with Asperger syndrome will not be able to process all the social information available at any given moment and the 'rapport' will be felt to be lacking or the interaction perceived as nothing so much as clumsy.

There are different levels of mentalising. The most basic level can be conceptualised in terms of the person understanding that 'I think that you think' (first level/first degree mental representation – or 'metarepresentations'). The next stage corresponds to 'I think that you think that she thinks' (second level mental representation). Further levels are self-evident ('I think that you think that she thinks that he thinks' etc.) and correspond to third and higher levels of metarepresentations. People with classic autism have difficulties already at the first level, and these problems usually persist throughout life. Individuals with Asperger syndrome appear to have such problems up until about age 4–6 years, after which problems at the second level may be obvious up until about 10 years of age when difficulties at the third or higher levels may be 'all' that remains. In other words: the ability underlying empathy skills is severely delayed in its development and may never reach the level attained by most 'typically developing' people before adolescence. Based on clinical work there can be no doubt that persons with Asperger syndrome find it tiresome and strenuous to reflect about other people's thoughts and feelings. It would not occur to them intuitively to consider other people's perspectives or to go outside their own circumscribed egocentric vantage point. Opinion is divided as to the specificity of mentalising problems in autism spectrum disorders. Several studies suggest that mild to moderate problems in the field of mentalising occur in a number of conditions, not just autism spectrum disorders. It is clear that a measure of mental, not least verbal, ability is required to pass theory of mind tasks, including those at the primary 'first level'. Although there are indications that typically developing children have emerging theory of mind skills already under age 1 year, in order to pass the formal mentalising tests, a mental age of 4–6 years would be required. This means that teenagers with severe mental retardation or children with major language problems cannot be expected to do well on such mentalising tests. Children diagnosed as suffering from attention-deficit/hyperactivity disorder (ADHD) or deficits in attention, motor control and perception (DAMP) who have marked autistic features, have mentalising problems that are strongly reminiscent of those encountered in classic autism. However, those with ADHD or DAMP who do not show marked autistic features may have no, or only minor, mentalising problems. Shared attention is considered by many to be one of the prerequisites for the development of a theory of mind. Shared attention refers to the capacity to look at an object or observe something going on 'together with' somebody else while being cognisant of the fact that the other person is observing the same thing. This ability can be observed in infants age 1 year pointing to a lamp, looking at it and then looking at mother to ascertain that she too is looking at the lamp: mother and child 'share attention'. Some researchers have posited that typically developing children have an innate ability to detect the gaze direction of other people. This ability will secure the development of a 'picture of the world' similar to that of important individuals in the close environment. A poorly developed gaze direction detector would be characteristic of people with autism spectrum disorders, including those with Asperger syndrome. If you are not attending to or looking at the same things or events as other people in your close environment, you will not have a good understanding of what other people find important or at which point other people would like to attract your attention. The basis for normal development of shared attention abilities will not be present. The ability to develop normal mentalising and empathy would therefore be seriously hampered.

Mentalising abilities require the optimal functioning of many different functional regions of the brain. Areas in the temporal, frontal and frontotemporal regions of the brain appear to be required for the emergence of 'normal' empathy skills. It is possible that optimal functions in a specific area in the left portion of the frontal lobe (Brodmann area 8/9) are necessary for the acquisition of adequate empathy skills. This brain area has been suggested to be crucially important for the ability to process mentalising tasks in a rapid and efficient manner.

Impaired mentalising can be inferred by poor results on certain neuro-psychological tests. Correct solutions to the more complex tasks of the Picture Arrangement subtests of the WISC-R (Wechsler Intelligence Scale for Children – Revised) and the WAIS-R (Wechsler Adult Intelligence Scale

– Revised) require some understanding of the thoughts, wishes and feelings of other people. Pictures depicting various types of events – ranging from very 'concrete' to rather more 'mental' – have to be arranged in order so as to produce a coherent 'story'. Individuals with Asperger syndrome, like the majority of those with autism, have considerable difficulty solving these tasks. They may pass the Picture Arrangement tasks that measure mechanistic understanding of an event but fail on those that require an understanding of the feelings and intentions of the people appearing in the pictures. The Picture Arrangement subtest of the WISC-III (a newer version than the WISC-R) appears to be considerably less efficient in tapping mentalising problems, possibly because there are more visual perceptual clues to the correct solution of the tasks on this version than that of the WISC-R. Simon Baron-Cohen has designed a series of Picture Arrangements specifically for use with individuals with autism spectrum disorders (Baron-Cohen et al. 1986).

The comprehension subtest of the various Wechsler scales can be seen as a measure of common sense. The proband is requested to respond to questions like: 'What would you do in case of a fire?' Verbal children with classic autism often have great difficulty with open questions of this kind and usually fail on this test. Young children with Asperger syndrome may also fall short of the mark on this test. However, as they grow older, they usually do well or even very well on the Comprehension test. Their verbal skills and the fact that people around them may have trained them specifically in commonsensical matters may gradually lead to 'concrete' knowledge regarding how one is expected to cope with a number of fairly predictable psychosocial situations. Parents or teachers may have understood intuitively that the young child with Asperger syndrome lacks common sense and may therefore have gone to considerable lengths to train the child in such skills.

There are a number of other tests that purport to tap mentalising deficits. Some of these have been widely used ('Sally–Anne', 'Smarties', 'Rabbit') and can be helpful in exploring theory of mind deficits in individuals with autism spectrum disorders. However, the psychometric properties for some of them have not been well explored. Many of these tests have been developed by research groups around Uta Frith, Simon Baron-Cohen and Francesca Happé. For older individuals on the autism spectrum there are more complex and subtle tests – including 'Strange stories' and tests of humour and irony – aiming to tap into the area of mentalising abilities. Some of these tests have been developed by Claire Hughes and Margaret Dewey (and the groups of researchers just referred to). Several studies have shown mentalising problems in groups of children who do not have autism or Asperger syndrome. Thus, theory of mind problems are not unique to autism spectrum disorders. Nevertheless, they are very common in such disorders. Understanding the implications of having theory of mind problems has opened a new window on autism and Asperger syndrome. Many of the social and communication problems typical of these conditions can be interpreted and effectively dealt with within the framework of mentalising deficits.

Factual memory, procedural learning and automatisation skills

Children with autism spectrum disorders without mental retardation usually have no or only relatively minor problems with factual knowledge, 'concrete' understanding of the world, or what, in the terminology of some cognitive psychologists, is referred to as 'folk physics'. Some results of neuropsychological studies suggest that, at least in respect of verbal memory, individuals with autism spectrum disorders including Asperger syndrome, may have better memory than other people. In particular, they appear to be better able to discriminate between true and false memories. This is an asset, but also represents a sign that semantic representations comprise a less distributed brain network in autism spectrum disorders.

In spite of these relative strengths in the field of factual knowledge, individuals with Asperger syndrome often have major problems learning procedures. Doing more than one thing at a time is difficult, and maintaining a strategy through a sequence of events is extremely difficult in real life settings, even when laboratory test results would suggest that there should be no difficulty.

Closely related to procedural learning is automatisation. Normal learning is characterised by learned material becoming more or less automatised after a period of training. The learned skill will then be retrieved in an automatic fashion whenever required. This retrieval ability, at least in matters of practical learning, is sometimes severely impaired in Asperger syndrome (and in DAMP). However, there are currently no generally agreed tests tapping into this area of functioning. Nevertheless, many tests of motor skills comprise repetitive activities and the automatisation problems usually become obvious during the performance of such tasks. Jumping up and down on one leg can be easy to do for somebody with Asperger syndrome, but often only for a few seconds. If the examiner does not 'support' the continued exercise by saying 'hop-hop-hop' or 'one-two-three', the child will just stop or fall out of the rhythm. Working memory deficits and attention problems may also contribute to problems in this domain. However, the ability to concentrate is usually not very much impaired in Asperger syndrome (on the contrary, it may be excellent, given the right situation and motivation), and attention dysfunction, therefore, does not appear to be a major factor in the 'automatisation problems'.

Executive functions

The ability to plan in order to attain a goal, to keep to a strategy for that purpose, keeping the goal, the strategy and sequence of events in 'working memory', and postponing the need for instant gratification, are all important components of the so-called 'executive function construct'. Executive functions can also be described as 'purposeful, future oriented activities'. The ability to conceive of a sequence of events, the order in which they occur and the ability to understand cause and effect are core aspects of executive functions. The sense of time is closely related to these. Some researchers would also include working memory (the ability to 'hold' information needed for problem solving 'in mind'), attention abilities and the capacity to control impulses among the executive functions, whereas others would treat these as separate components.

It has now been well documented that individuals with Asperger syndrome have considerable problems with executive functions, including, in certain cases, some aspects of working memory, attention, and impulse control. It also seems clear that these problems are responsible for many of the everyday functional impairments shown by people with high-functioning autism spectrum disorders. What is much less well understood is how specific these problems are. Several studies have demonstrated 'executive function deficits' in a variety of child neuropsychiatric syndromes, including ADHD and DAMP. The ability to plan ahead, motivation, sequencing and time concepts are often poorly developed in these conditions just as they are in Asperger syndrome. The poor concept of time and the slowness of some individuals with Asperger syndrome can be one of their most, sometimes *the* most, handicapping problems.

Clinical experience suggests that executive dysfunction in Asperger syndrome tends to predict a poor outcome as regards education and psychosocial adjustment. In cases with such dysfunction, it is very important to provide external structure in the educational setting, so as to compensate for poor inner structuring skills, and to avoid the chaos which otherwise tends to develop in the life of a person with Asperger syndrome.

Executive functions are, almost by tradition, considered to be largely located in the prefrontal areas of the frontal lobes of the brain. For a long time, researchers believed that these areas were functionally relatively inactive well into the school years. Recent studies have shown that many executive functions – including the ability to control impulses – are in operation already around 1 year of age. As already mentioned, frontal areas of the brain appear to be functionally impaired or different in Asperger syndrome.

The common Wechsler scales of intelligence (WISC, WAIS) include subtests that reflect executive functions. Coding and Arithmetic are examples of such subtests. Many individuals with Asperger syndrome, just like those with ADHD/DAMP fail or perform less well on these. The Wisconsin Card Sorting Test, in which the proband is required to stay with or change strategy according to the implicit information given by the examiner, is another commonly used test of executive functions. Individuals with Asperger syndrome often have problems with this test. There are also so-called Go/No Go and Conflict tests (both auditory and visual), during which the child is requested to react to a stimulus and also to inhibit reactions to stimuli. Children with Asperger syndrome again score poorly on certain aspects of these tests, much along the lines of those with ADHD/DAMP.

Central coherence

Seeing beyond detail and grasping the 'big picture' can be terribly difficult for individuals in the autism spectrum. The laboratory results regarding certain aspects of central coherence in Asperger syndrome have been rather conflicting, some studies suggesting severe problems in this domain, whereas others have found only minor or no deviations from the norm.

Nevertheless, clinical experience abounds with real-life examples of how people with Asperger syndrome become overfixated on detail and fail to fit them together to something 'whole'. There are instances when it can be helpful to fixate on details, but there are obvious problems connected with inability to 'see the wood for all the trees'. One of my patients has a fantastic ability to describe the features of other people's faces, bodies, clothes and shoes out of his memory. However, he is completely lost when asked to identify these people from photographs or in a 'face-to-face' real life setting.

In the WISC and WAIS tests there are two subtests, Block Design and Object Assembly, that can help tap problems in the field of visual central coherence. The Object Assembly test consists of cardboard pieces of a puzzle outlining a horse, hand etc. For anybody with a good sense of 'wholes' it is easy to see what they represent, but for somebody with a fixation on detail, this test can be extremely difficult. Quite a number of those with Asperger syndrome do poorly on this test. On the Block Design test, on the contrary, the individual is helped by not being distracted by 'the whole picture'. People with autism spectrum disorders often do very well on this subtest. A combination of good results on the Block Design subtest and poorer results on the Object Assembly is very common in Asperger syndrome.

'Intelligence'

People with Asperger syndrome are often of high intelligence. However, this statement needs to be tempered by the fact that their IQ test results are usually uneven, with major peaks and troughs. The troughs, often in areas reflecting executive function and central coherence problems can contribute to relatively severe learning problems. The fact that so many people with Asperger syndrome become bored whenever required to do things for which they were not originally motivated further contributes to the inability to make good use of the high intelligence.

Verbal intelligence is often, though by no means always, better than so-called performance intelligence. The discrepancy between verbal IQ and performance IQ can be very marked (25 points difference or more). I have some patients who have a verbal IQ of 130 and a performance IQ of around

70. This, in other words, is then a person of superior intelligence in the verbal field and yet bordering on mental retardation in the performance field. It is not difficult to imagine that such discrepancies can be difficult to live with ('Who am I? Am I a genius or just plain stupid?'). They also contribute to other people making severe mistakes in their personal judgements and therefore making unreasonable demands ('He must do this task! Somebody with such excellent verbal skills must be highly intelligent and be able to live up to my simple demands!'). These huge discrepancies between verbal and performance IQ are sometimes referred to as 'non-verbal learning disability'. Even though it is not exceptional for the discrepancy to run in the other direction (i.e. performance IQ much greater than verbal IQ), there is no corresponding 'label' for that condition. Individuals with this latter pattern, because of their rather poor verbal skills are often believed to be much more 'stupid' than they actually are.

One of the greatest assets of many people with Asperger syndrome is their high intelligence. It is therefore sad to see sometimes how a young adult person with an IQ of over 150 can be completely lost in education settings where there is little outer structure. One of my patients with such a high IQ did well during the school years when the structures surrounding him were almost rigid and school work was checked on every day. At university he has failed completely, mostly because he has been expected to motivate himself and structure his work all by himself.

Concluding remarks

Individuals with Asperger syndrome usually have problems with executive functions, mentalising and procedural learning/automatisation. They often have problems with central coherence also. They are, on average, slow in their problem-solving style. No highly specific neuropsychological or cognitive psychological deficit has yet been demonstrated in autism spectrum disorders. Rather, it is the pattern of the deficits that is characteristic. There are a number of tests available that can help home in on the cognitive difficulties and the particular cognitive style of people with Asperger syndrome. Among these, some of the old and much used instruments, such as the WISC and the WAIS, are still very helpful tools in the diagnostic process.

Diagnosis and work-up

Many individuals with Asperger syndrome present to childhood services including child and adolescent psychiatric clinics, child guidance clinics and paediatric clinics. Other children and adolescents come to the attention of GPs, developmental paediatricians, neurologists or neuropsychiatrists, or even clinical geneticists. Some, though not all, of these will be correctly identified and diagnosed as having an autism spectrum disorder/Asperger syndrome. Increasing numbers who were never diagnosed in childhood – or who received other, less informative diagnoses – apply for help in adult psychiatric clinics.

All people with Asperger syndrome and marked psychosocial adaptation problems should be examined by a medical doctor with training in autism spectrum disorders. In addition, there is usually a need for assessment by a psychologist with specific knowledge in the field.

Occasionally there is a need for further medical work-up, including brain imaging, EEG, blood – including genetic – and urine tests.

Assessment by a skilled special education teacher is also often required, particularly in the case of school-age children.

Medical assessment

The medical doctor will have to review the individual's early developmental history with the mother or some other person who knew the patient well when he was of preschool age. It is essential that the doctor is familiar with the symptoms and course of autism spectrum disorders and other child neuropsychiatric problems. The ability to conduct a proper 'developmental interview' is dependent on specific knowledge and clinical experience in the field. Current symptoms and problems are, of course, also very important to assess, but it is the early history which will usually determine whether a diagnosis of an autism spectrum disorder/Asperger syndrome applies or not.

Once the doctor suspects that the patient may indeed have Asperger syndrome, it is often helpful to give out some written material about high-functioning autism/Asperger syndrome to those that have provided the information that formed the basis for the clinical suspicion. Arranging for an early return visit and asking the informant(s) to read the material and make notes as to the relevance of the characteristics of the syndrome in the particular case under consideration is often indicated.

The patient himself/herself, of course, has to be meticulously physically and psychiatrically examined (including a neuromotor and neurological examination), even in cases presenting with the classical symptoms. It is not uncommon for a very experienced clinician to be able to make a relatively definitive diagnosis after having spent only a quarter of an hour with the patient. The peculiar way of avoiding gaze contact coupled with the odd staring fixation at other times, the formal yet naïve approach, the monotone voice with its characteristic shrillness, the limited amount of gesture and the immediate insistence on 'discussing' or lecturing about a favourite topic – all of these can be so characteristic that it immediately becomes clear that no diagnosis other than Asperger syndrome can apply. More rarely, it may be very difficult to arrive at a correct diagnosis, and the physician may have to arrange to meet the individual several times for several hours until he/she feels convinced of the diagnosis or that it does not apply. Differential diagnosis may be particularly difficult in girls and women, in patients who receive neuroleptic medication, in adults who have a long history of adult psychiatric problems and hence a list of psychiatric diagnoses, inappropriate treatments (including group psychotherapy and unusual medications), a prior history of eating disorder or alcoholism.

The examining doctor may want to use an interview schedule specifically designed for high-functioning autism or Asperger syndrome. In individuals who do not appear to be intellectually bright, the CARS (Childhood Autism Rating Scale) developed by Eric Schopler and his group in North Carolina – may be helpful in delineating the scope and type of problems. For those with higher IQ, the CARS is usually inappropriate. The ASDI (Asperger Syndrome and High-functioning Autism Diagnostic Interview), developed by my own group (see Appendix I), covering the 20 symptom areas included as diagnostic criteria for the disorder according to Gillberg (Gillberg et al. 2001), can be helpful in such cases. The ASSQ (Asperger Syndrome and other autism spectrum disorders Screening Questionnaire) (Ehlers and Gillberg 1993) and the ASDASQ (Autism Spectrum Disorders in Adults Screening Questionnaire) (Nylander and Gillberg 2001), also developed by my group (see Appendix II and III), may be useful screening devices for relatives and staff but cannot be used as diagnostic instruments. The ASSQ contains 27 items and the ASDASQ contains 9 simple questions. The total range of scores is 0–54 on the ASSQ and 0–9 on the ASDASQ. Scores of about 20 or above on the ASSQ (teacher or parent) and 6 or more on the ASDASQ (staff in adult psychiatric services) should alert the clinician to the very likely possibility that the patient may be suffering from an autism spectrum disorder.

The DISCO (Diagnosis of Social and Communication Disorders), developed by Lorna Wing and Judy Gould in London (Wing et al. 2001), is a 2–3 hour interview which covers all the relevant symptom areas in depth. It should be used with an informant who knew the individual with suspected Asperger syndrome when he/she was young (much of the content of the interview is related to the early development of the child). It can be extremely useful when diagnosis is in doubt, for research purposes, or in patients for whom it becomes clear at an early stage that long-term habilitation measures will be required. The few hours spent on the interview with a relative of the patient are usually a good investment, not only because it allows for more fine-grained diagnosis, but also because it can work a a 'therapeutic session'. A mother or father reviewing their child's early development and current problems will often find it very helpful to analyse the situation in the 'coherent context' of an autism spectrum disorder. Sometimes, it is only during an interview of this kind that the parent feels she/he 'understood what it was all about, finally seeing the bits and pieces fall into place'.

The ADI-R (Autism Diagnostic Interview Revised), developed by Michael Rutter and his group in London, is perhaps more appropriate for research purposes and for lower-functioning individuals in the autism spectrum (Lord et al. 1994). Both the ADI-R and the DISCO require prior training courses before they can be used in clinical or research practice.

Tourette syndrome or other tic disorders are common in Asperger syndrome. The same holds for ADHD (and DAMP) symptoms. Catatonic features and other motor disorders occur in a substantial minority of cases. The examining doctor will need to screen for these disorders and, whenever a suspicion is raised, probe into these diagnostic categories in a systematic fashion.

Hearing and vision are usually normal in Asperger syndrome, but quite a proportion of affected individuals have visual and/or hearing problems. Visual and hearing screens are indicated in all cases, and the threshold for referring on to an ophthalmologist or audiologist should be low. Having reduced vision or hearing could seriously compromise development even in very high-functioning individuals with Asperger syndrome, who may appear to be of subnormal intelligence or mentally retarded if left undiagnosed and unattended to.

It is not extremely rare, although by no means common, for another medical disorder to underlie Asperger syndrome. Such disorders may be chromosomal/genetic (such as in fragile X syndrome, 22q11-deletion syndrome, or tuberous sclerosis) or acquired (such as in foetal alcohol syndrome or syndromes attributed to specific medications in utero). The examining doctor has to have sufficient knowledge about the possible underlying factors so as to be able to determine which, if any, additional laboratory or other tests will have to be performed. These may include an EEG, a brain imaging examination procedure, or a chromosomal – or otherwise genetic – test (see further below, p. 93).

Psychological assessment

Every person seeking help and raising suspicions of suffering from Asperger syndrome should be given a cognitive test. The previously mentioned Wechsler scales (WISC, WAIS for example) are especially useful. The Wechsler scales often yield a characteristic profile with good or even superior results on subtests of 'information', 'comprehension', 'vocabulary' and 'similarities', and less good or markedly inferior results on subtests of 'object assembly', 'arithmetic', 'coding' and 'picture arrangement'. This profile is similar to that encountered in the syndrome of DAMP (deficits in attention, motor control and perception), except as regards picture arrangement, low results on which subtest (at least on the WISC-R and WAIS-R, probably not the WISC-III) is typical of autism. This can also be expressed as Asperger individuals having good skills in verbal domains, while at the same time functioning much less well in areas of visual perception. The neuropsychological test results are also reminiscent of those encountered in the syndrome of non-verbal learning disorder.

It is often helpful to perform other neuropsychological tests tapping attentional, memory, planning, central coherence and theory of mind functions as well as reaction times and overall speed. This may be especially important in young adult individuals who may need guidance in respect of finding the most appropriate education and/or work. Such tests should be performed after a thorough review of the need for specific interventions, and are not generally needed as part of the work-up for the diagnosis of Asperger syndrome in itself.

Other evaluations and tests

Additional medical examinations are sometimes required. This is especially the case if the patient with Asperger syndrome has a learning disorder or an IQ which is in the subaverage range. However, it should not be presumed that all individuals with normal or superior IQ are in need of no further medical examinations. A chromosomal analysis is indicated when the physical appearance (including abnormal tallness) suggests the presence of a specific chromosomal disorder (including an aberrant number of sex chromosomes). Specific DNA tests (e.g. for the fragile X syndrome, the 22q11-deletion syndrome and Williams syndrome) are required in cases with a history and symptoms suggesting underlying specific genetic disorders. An EEG can be helpful in differential diagnosis of patients with 'staring spells', 'vacant gaze behaviours', paroxysmal episodes of unaccountable and/or bizarre behaviours, or in patients with severely disturbed sleep patterns. An MRI (functional magnetic resonance imaging) of the brain is sometimes indicated to rule out/rule in specific conditions. However, at the present stage of our knowledge, MRI or other brain imaging techniques should not be considered routine in the work-up of individuals with Asperger syndrome. A range of other examinations – including blood, urine and, occasionally, cerebrospinal fluid sampling – may be required if the clinical examination raises the suspicion of a metabolic/neurometabolic disorder. Full coverage of the many possibilities that need to be considered in individuals with autism spectrum disorders is beyond the scope of this book. A comprehensive review with practical guidelines is provided in *The Biology of the Autistic Syndromes*, by Gillberg and Coleman (2000).

Concluding remarks

The work-up in cases of Asperger syndrome can usually be relatively restricted. Some things are always required though: a physical examination (including hearing and vision tests in all cases), a full medical and psychiatric history and a psychological assessment. Other analyses, such as chromosome tests, DNA tests, MRI and EEG are required only in certain cases. It is the autism expert doctor's task to review all the available data and make a clinical judgement as to what is required in terms of additional laboratory evaluations.

Outcome in the longer term: adults with Asperger syndrome

Outcome in Asperger syndrome is very variable. Many of those with a characteristic pattern of problems in childhood are functioning well in adult age, even though the personality traits that were evident early on tend to be highly persistent. Others have a very poor prognosis from the psycho-social adjustment point of view and cannot manage independently in adult life. Others function along a spectrum in between excellent and highly restricted outcomes.

It is still much too early to determine how large a proportion of those with the childhood presentation of Asperger syndrome will fall into any one of the three adult outcome groups. So far, no longitudinal prospective studies of representative cases of the syndrome have been published. It is only when the results of such studies are available that we will know the answer to the question: What is the natural course of Asperger syndrome in the general population?

The basic problems

In spite of the lack of systematic empirical studies, there is a wealth of clinical experience which forms a fairly sound basis for conclusions about certain aspects of longer-term outcome in Asperger syndrome.

Virtually all authors in the field seem to be agreed that the basic and characteristic social, communicative and behavioural/imagination problems encountered in Asperger syndrome are likely to persist throughout life. Even when the symptoms become modified and the clinical picture is muddled by associated problems of various kinds (including alcoholism, confusional states, depression and fixation on death themes), the specific inability to react swiftly and interact intuitively in social and flexible ways with other people will persist. This can be felt as an almost complete lack of 'natural improvisation' skills. Some individuals with the syndrome may be able to imitate a number of social 'roles' and to 'act' such roles for a limited amount of time, sometimes almost to perfection. This will almost definitely fool those not well aware of the basic problems, and the person with Asperger syndrome may appear completely 'normal', at least for a brief period of time. However, the deficient improvisation skills will usually become evident very soon. Rigidity, dependence on routines and lack of social common sense will usually remain 'unperturbed' by experience, life events, and, for that matter, various forms of therapy.

The aloof group

In my experience, at least two out of every five individuals with Asperger syndrome will remain withdrawn and aloof in adult age. They lead an isolated life and have difficulty managing or even tolerating the company of other people. They will choose isolation whenever possible. A limited number of this group may actually get married and have children, but it is their spouse who takes care of all kinds of social interaction. They will withdraw to their room or 'quarters' as soon as dinner has been finished and will not want to waste time on trivial matters such as small-talk or disquisitions about minor everyday things. Contrary to other people their time at the working desk or in their favourite chair is spent on 'important things' or 'this and that'. This may infer that they are actually working on a project of sorts, but it might just as well involve time running away while they 'sit and think' or are 'busy with philosophical matters'. On direct questioning it may become clear that they do not, in fact, sit around and think, but that they feel their head is all 'empty'.

A small subgroup among the withdrawn group of adults with Asperger syndrome is constituted by those who actually would be best characterised as having classic autism. They appear to be living in a world completely their own, and appear not be listening when other people speak to them. They may only react when hands are clapped together or their name is being literally shouted at them. For a few seconds their attention may be attracted only to sink back into an oblivious, withdrawn attitude. Adult psychiatrists often think of this subgroup as having 'chronic but atypical depression', 'schizophreniform disorder' or 'type II schizophrenia'.

Just as in the other groups (the active group and the passive group, see below), some of the withdrawn individuals with Asperger syndrome are perceived as distant, cold, mean or hard. Others may evoke very different feelings and opinions: childish, naïve, heart-breaking, strange, serene, odd or old-fashioned.

The active and odd group

Some, perhaps one in five (or even two in five) of all with Asperger syndrome, belong in a group which is very active (and sometimes very successful in that activity), but with a tendency to do and say very odd things in social settings. They may be lacking in distance and reticence and show little or no feeling for other people. They may speak in a loud voice when a whisper is what is expected. They tend to stare and to make demands with no sign of embarrassment. They will go on at length about their special interest, not noticing other people's reactions or even the falling asleep of a conversation partner. They may be thought of as 'chauvinists' or 'nerds'. Some will have a very high tempo and may be thought of as manic. Just occasionally they may wind themselves up to the level of true 'mania' and may even be admitted to a psychiatric clinic under just such a diagnosis (which, incidentally, may sometimes be absolutely right; there is probably a marked overrepresentation of manic-depressive illness in individuals with Asperger syndrome). Others will be perceived as well-meaning and yet be thought of as tiresome and frustrating.

The passive group

A rather smaller group of all those who showed the symptoms of Asperger syndrome in childhood develop a passive 'personality' later in life. Such individuals may be extremely difficult to recognise as having the syndrome if you did not know them when they were much younger. They make little 'fuss', and lead a withdrawn life without rejecting other people. They do not take initiatives to broaden their group of peers or to 'make an impression'.

It is only when you get to know them in a more personal way that the typical Asperger personality will 'let on'. Under the friendly, superficially unobtrusive surface resides a rigid, stiff, obsessional, greedy and, quite often, overvaluing attitude. They may be perceived as 'obsessive–compulsive' or 'passive-aggressive'. It is particularly among these individuals with Asperger syndrome that one encounters those who will be described as 'good', 'kind' even 'saintly', even though some of them will come across as covertly negativistic. Long-term experience with this group will reveal that 'unfeeling' criticism and negative fixation on certain themes or people may underlie the 'friendly' attitude. I know a few people with Asperger syndrome who have this type of outcome ('passive/friendly') who have actually persecuted other people.

Other problems

There is probably a marked overrepresentation of drug and alcohol abuse, depression, obsessive–compulsive symptoms, fixation on death themes, suicidal thoughts and suicide in Asperger syndrome.

It now seems likely that many individuals with childhood onset symptoms of Asperger syndrome apply for adult psychiatric help without having consulted psychiatric services in childhood or adolescence, and hence being 'without an appropriate diagnosis'. Such individuals will almost invariably receive a very different diagnosis by the attending adult psychiatrist. The most common among such diagnoses may be: 'personality disorder' (obsessive–compulsive, paranoid, schizoid, schizotypal, avoidant and borderline, in particular), 'schizophrenia or schizophreniform psychosis', 'unspecified psychosis' or 'affective disorder'. I have also met many who have presented in adult age with alcoholism, other drug abuse, odd criminal behaviours, dramatic rage or aggressive behaviours, social phobia or confusional states occurring in circumstances of stress (which will usually be perceived by other people as 'mild' or even 'non-existent'). Individuals with Asperger syndrome thus diagnosed often receive treatment with neuroleptic or other medications which often give little benefit and sometimes cause serious side effects.

An appropriate diagnosis of Asperger syndrome can often be made on the basis of a combination of (i) in-depth interviews with those who knew the individual during the preschool and early school age years, and (ii) personal clinical examination and interview of the individual suspected of suffering from Asperger syndrome. The diagnosis can be made with a fair degree of confidence even when the individual is age 20 years or more. However, it does require a considerable degree of clinical know-how and experience on the part of the examining doctor. Therefore, all psychiatrists need to have specific training in the field of autism spectrum disorders, if adults with autism spectrum disorders are to receive adequate diagnosis and work-up in the future.

Concluding remarks

Outcome in Asperger syndrome is very variable. Many with the disorder do well as adults and may attain status as leaders in their particular field. However, the vast majority are characterised by continued restriction of reciprocal social interaction and various repetitive/ritualistic behaviours. Some develop severe psychiatric problems. There is a considerable risk that such problems may be misinterpreted and treated in less than helpful ways. Better knowledge about Asperger syndrome and other high-functioning autism spectrum disorders among specialists in adult services is likely to provide the best remedy for such mistakes.

Attitudes, interventions and treatment

The single most important intervention when it comes to improving the quality of life of individuals with Asperger syndrome and their families is the attempt to change people's attitudes, both as regards the specific problems and their nature and the people affected. Such a change of attitude cannot take place without a proper diagnosis.

It is often necessary to intervene in one way or another in the school setting or at work. This, to a considerable extent, has to do with information and spreading of knowledge about the impairments associated with Asperger syndrome. Sometimes, indeed quite often, other measures will be required. There is no general need for 'treatment' of the fundamental traits associated with the syndrome as such, at least not at the present stage of our knowledge. There is no 'cure' for the basic problems, and, once the diagnosis is made, many do not feel the need for treatment of any kind. Nevertheless, interventions that include educational and psychological support, are often extremely helpful and should always be considered once the diagnosis has been made. Psychoeducational measures, systematic training of skills, individual talks with somebody knowledgeable about Asperger syndrome, and, occasionally, medication, may all be required in individual cases.

General aspects

Respect for the individual with Asperger syndrome must always take precedence in the planning of help and treatment for people with this variant of autism spectrum disorder. In spite of many superficial similarities, people with Asperger syndrome are all different, and there are no two people with the diagnosis who benefit from exactly the same kind of intervention approaches. As with other people, there is considerable variation in respect of the general intellectual level. The most highly intelligent are, of course, much better at abstractions than those who are of low normal intelligence. (Even so, there is usually a quality of 'concreteness' in people with Asperger syndrome, quite regardless of the overall level of IQ.) An intervention programme identical for all with the syndrome, be it psychological, educational or medical/pharmacological, should never be attempted.

Most people with Asperger syndrome have a type of humour that differs from that of people in general. Some appear to be totally devoid of humour, always serious and may be thought of as 'deep', 'moody', 'dysphoric' or constantly 'brooding'. They may occasionally laugh, for instance on hearing a word game or a particularly fancy rhyme, but may be notorious for their failure to ever smile. Others love to play around with words and statements made by famous people or to draw attention to the many absurdities of life. Quite a few will be extremely amused by things that would be perceived by other people as tragic, cynical or just plain evil. It is often impossible to get them to explain what it is that is so funny. They may come up with convoluted explanations or just look at the other person with a shrug of the shoulders to indicate, 'You must be such a fool not to understand the hilariousness of this.' There are those who are completely thrown by slap-stick humour and pranks. I know several 'comedians' who will tell little anecdotes and funny jokes as soon as an opportunity presents itself (and sometimes even when it does not). The problem in such cases arises when teachers, peers or relatives take the opportunity of themselves telling a joke. Quite unexpectedly, at least if you are not familiar with the diagnosis of Asperger syndrome and its applications, this joke may be completely mis-construed and interpreted in a negative way and form the underpinnings of a row. It is only when another person is very well acquainted with 'Asperger humour' in general and the individual's interests and attitudes in particular, that trying to strike a common chord and be funny, can be recommended at all.

People with Asperger syndrome are often very good observers and can make astute remarks about other people's behaviours and appearance. To the contrary, the vast majority cannot support even the slightest hint of similar remarks made with reference to themselves by other people. In fact, they may oppose any kind of remark about their own behaviour made by others, and it tends to make little difference if strangers or well-known people are involved. It is sometimes unbelievably easy to inadvertently offend a person with Asperger syndrome. Feelings of being 'miffed', 'slighted', 'devastated', 'belittled', 'crushed', 'slandered' or 'back-stabbed' are commonplace reactions to other people having said anything personal at all. Something that was said is being interpreted in a concrete way to mean something very different from what was originally intended. It may be impossible to ever repair the damage and make things right after such a 'blunder'. This may make it very difficult to judge whether bullying has indeed occurred. This is an especially relevant issue, given that bullying is very common in Asperger syndrome. Nevertheless, it has to be said that, just occasionally, one might get very close to a person with Asperger syndrome if one learns to understand the special sense of humour which is his/her hallmark and which may be perceived by other people as odd, strange or black.

People with Asperger syndrome often benefit, and like it, if approached 'in a concrete manner'. Just as they themselves perceive of the world and other people in concrete ways – even if they may be using complex, intricate and elaborate language – so would they want other people to interact with them in everyday situations. Many are those who become confused when other people want to share gossip, secrets, or speak at length about social relationships, 'hunches' and 'feelings'. Some of the more talented people with the syndrome may take some degree of pleasure in (or may even be obsessed with) collecting facts about other people, and may occasionally come across as gossipy. As soon as other people take them up on the issue and want to discuss these interesting individuals who seem to interest them so deeply and want to talk about their ideas, thoughts and feelings, they appear to lose all interest in the matter. Their gaze goes blank and they may start talking about something completely different. Alternatively, they may become extremely anxious and start looking around for a way to escape. One is usually better off on neutral ground, i.e. matters related to concrete fact or issues that are 'unequivocal'.

It is of great importance to provide straightforward information. The fewer the complications in the message delivered the better. Do not engage in cumbersome phrases, convoluted questions, hints, hidden meanings or overly polite communications. It is usually much better to come forth and 'say it straight', avoiding, as far as possible, all risk of misinterpretation. With some individuals it would be impossible to communicate the underlying message by saying: 'Could you open the window?' (which might lead to a 'Yes' response without any action being taken; the individual responding to the concrete question whether he/she *has the ability to open the window*), whereas 'Open the window!' would lead to the desired activity. Unfortunately, it is not uncommon for people not acquainted with the underlying problems in Asperger syndrome, to react negatively to such a 'harsh' communication style, which may be employed by relatives, teachers and friends, who through years of trial and error have found this method to be 'the only road to understanding'.

Being presented with options, at least if unprepared, is often a cause for extreme concern, anguish and even panic for a person with Asperger syndrome. He/she will often have great difficulty imagining what the various choices really are or represent, and so become confused and anxious. It is usually much better either to present just one alternative and ask a 'yes'/'no' question or even to suggest that 'this is going to be the best choice' (providing, of course, that the person presenting the choice, knows the individual with Asperger syndrome very well). It is only after many trials of successful suggestions of this kind (i.e. when the person with Asperger syndrome has experienced first-hand that the proposed choice was really a good one) that one should try and introduce – slowly, gradually – more complicated choice situations.

As should have become clear from the foregoing, it is often only when people know about the fundamentals of Asperger syndrome and have in-depth knowledge about the individual with the diagnosis that they can provide a good environment that does not cause concern, anxiety or extreme stress. This is one of the reasons why it is of the utmost importance that people with Asperger syndrome are surrounded – in all important situations and at all stages of development (childhood, adolescence and adult age) – by a small group of people who *really know* them.

A high degree of structure, order and predictability, both at school/work and at home/during leisure time are usually prerequisites for a good quality of life for individuals with Asperger syndrome. This is often true even in cases when at first glance clear structuring along these lines appears to be superfluous. Many people with the syndrome appear to be 'lazy', 'lacking in energy', 'chronically tired', or are constantly complaining about all the boring aspects of life. They may say no to all tasks that are presented without any prior preparation. Much of this behaviour is reminiscent of the kinds of problems encountered in the DAMP syndrome and ADHD (see chapter 3), and, indeed in any disorder reflecting underlying problems with executive functions. Providing 'external' executive functions (motivation, planning, structuring, sequencing and timing) when 'internal' ones are lacking or deficient seems like a rather obvious approach. A structured, indeed sometimes rather rigid, curriculum for the various activities of the day, is what usually works best. This is also what often works best with individuals who suffer from classic autism. However, by and large, for teachers and relatives it is much more difficult to appreciate this need in Asperger syndrome than in the more typical variants of autism, particularly in cases with superior intelligence.

A fundamental principle in all contacts with individuals with Asperger syndrome is the need to consider the possibility that what works best for oneself does not necessarily work at all for those with the disorder. Almost automatically, people will suggest interventions rooted in the formula: 'What works for me will work for other people.' This may be a completely mistaken view in Asperger syndrome. Instead, one needs to base suggestions for help in knowledge about the basic problems in Asperger syndrome after having listened respectfully to the person with that diagnosis. Things that may be felt to be extremely monotonous, boring or childish to somebody without the syndrome, may be thought of as very positive and interesting by the person with the disorder. As long as the activities that the person with Asperger syndrome engages in are not harmful or driven across all reasonable borders or repeated to the extent that learning and psychosocial adaptation are severely affected, people who 'want to help' should refrain from comparisons with themselves or other so-called normal people. It is important not to make judgements, rate activities or send the message that some activities are of higher quality than others. For instance, it may even be detrimental to suggest that socialising with other people always is to be preferred over performing a task in a meticulous and perfect manner.

Occasionally, the special interest patterns seen in Asperger syndrome can contribute to major problems. Some individuals are drawn to philosophy, religion, mysticism, occultism, sects (including with racial overtones) or other dogmatic movements. This can become very troublesome, not least because the person with Asperger syndrome may have greater difficulty than other people in keeping their distance from the subject matter. They may easily become completely obsessed and pursue an interest which, if not treated 'objectively' could soon lead to dangerous activities. Such interest patterns can, rarely, have positive connotations and inspire growth and helpful developments. For the most part, however, with hindsight, one wishes that one would have been able to prevent the development of such an obsessive interest in a 'dubious' area.

Perhaps the most difficult problem arises when the person with Asperger syndrome starts to show an interest in areas that touch on, or actually directly involve, violence. Weapons, poison, dynamite, sports with 'violent ingredients' (such as boxing or karate) can be tempting to some people with the syndrome. It is almost always advisable to try and distract interest from such potentially dangerous activities. Anyone who has major difficulties appreciating other people's thoughts, experiences and feelings runs a greatly increased risk of hurting (whether unintentionally or not) other people in the pursuit of such interests.

Nevertheless, it needs to be emphasised that people with Asperger syndrome are not at greatly increased risk of being involved in violent or criminal activities. The vast majority are strongly opposed to such actions: 'couldn't harm a fly' is a commonly heard description that is well suited to many people with Asperger syndrome.

Early and correct diagnosis: the impact of assessment

All individuals with Asperger syndrome symptoms who have serious problems in the field of psychosocial adaptation need a competent diagnostic work-up. Conversely, there is no need for such work-up in cases with good psychosocial adjustment. Maybe as many as half of all people who meet *symptom criteria* for Asperger syndrome have a reasonably acceptable life situation and neither they themselves, nor their relatives find reason to consult anyone about these *symptoms*. In such cases there is usually no need to try to prompt a diagnosis. However, in a subgroup, there may actually be major problems which the individuals themselves – or their parents – do not appreciate or refuse to admit. It could be a primary school child whose problems may be thought to be major by the class teacher – to the extent that it may actually be impossible to teach the child anything – but whose parents claim there is nothing 'wrong'. In such cases it is often necessary to allow plenty of time in order to try and convince the parents that the child is in need of help and therefore in need of a competent diagnostic work-up. Some fathers, and, albeit more rarely, mothers, who themselves have Asperger syndrome or marked autistic traits may feel that teachers exaggerate or that the school health officers or school psychologist tend to miss the point: just look at how well the parent who never received a diagnosis has done! It is sometimes possible through close contact with the family to convince them of the need for a comprehensive work-up. On other occasions, one may have to 'give up', realising, perhaps, that the parent may be quite right and that a diagnosis actually would not benefit the child in the given situation. There are, of course, also those cases in which a diagnosis is never made, and in which the failure to achieve this can have tragic consequences for the child, or cause major problems many years later when erroneous diagnoses of personality disorder or schizophrenia are made.

By and large, the diagnosis of Asperger syndrome is considered to be a great help in and of itself to the person affected, his family, other relatives, and for teachers and age peers. Many who have wondered over the years why so many things around them 'went wrong', find in the diagnosis itself the beginning of an explanation of so many difficulties that previously seemed to be incomprehensible. Reading about Asperger syndrome in a booklet, a book, or on the Internet can serve as an unexpected eye-opener, indeed quite often as a kind of positive revelation. The insight that there are others with similar, almost identical, problems is often an enormous relief. Parents, brothers, sisters and others close to the person affected, may find that having a name for the 'problem' makes them want to understand, change their attitudes and be constructive. Rather than being burdened by the diagnosis, the diagnosis itself takes a load off everybody involved. It paves the way for much more helpful attitudes and makes it possible to go on without constantly looking back, 'digging' hopelessly for more or less plausible explanations.

Attitudes

For people with neuropsychiatric problems, societal attitudes are of paramount importance when it comes to creating optimal conditions for the realisation of each individual's potential. This holds for Asperger syndrome as well as for those with more classical variants of autism. Disseminating knowledge through books, information leaflets, newspaper articles, radio, TV and the Internet are all essential elements in attempts to change the attitudes of other people. Education of teachers, psychologists, sociologists, doctors and other staff within the health and care systems is a prerequisite for enduring effects. The basic curriculum for the education of these categories should include state-of-the-art information about autism and Asperger syndrome. It is only when those who meet the individual with Asperger syndrome in their everyday life have sufficient knowledge about the basic impairments, that an environment can be created/adjusted so as not to be overly stressful to the person affected.

In the direct work with patients seeking help within the health service system, attempts to increase knowledge about Asperger syndrome, and change attitudes, are the backbone of all interventions. Without insight into the basic impairments and an approach that takes account of the problems associated with them, there is little that can be done to improve the situation at hand. Education, social skills training, other training (including physical), behaviour modification and medication all take a secondary role. The primary goal is to adjust the attitudes of other people (and to some extent that of the person with the disorder), and hence their interactions with and demands/expectations on the individual with Asperger syndrome. The 'hidden' functional impairments are usually much greater than appreciated by those who are not informed about the nature of the disorder.

School interventions

The level of knowledge has to be increased in schools and places where people with Asperger syndrome work. School health staff and doctors and nurses working in company health care systems have an important educational role in this context. They can – and should – work actively to spread general knowledge about autism spectrum disorders and ensure that people with probable Asperger syndrome if in need of help are referred for adequate work-up and possible interventions.

Psychoeducation

Psychoeducation measures are both general and specific. General measures are such interventions that aim to increase knowledge about a functional impairment – such as Asperger syndrome – among the public. Specific measures pertain to the individual and refer to the concerted attempts to raise the level of knowledge and optimise the educational and vocational interventions directed at him/her.

Some of the most intelligent children with Asperger syndrome can, and usually should, have their education in the setting of a 'normal' classroom, including, in some cases, a classroom with many pupils. In most cases, it is, however, important to make certain that the teachers are aware of the affected individual's diagnosis and its meaning. A high degree of structure is usually required. Expectations and demands that really correspond to the child's overall – and specific – level of functioning are crucial. It is not uncommon for demands to be much too low in some areas, while in others – particularly those that require social interaction, such as work in groups and the like – they may be unrealistically high. Close collaboration between children, parents and teachers, sometimes supported by the team of school health officers (doctor, psychologist, school nurse), is usually necessary in order to avoid major problems in school.

A smaller group of those with very high intelligence, a rather larger group of those with normal levels of intelligence, and virtually all of those with subnormal intelligence, will benefit from attending smaller classroom groups, perhaps containing no more than 6–15 pupils. Such groups might well comprise of individuals with similar problems, children with other neuropsychiatric disorders, so-called normal children with high intelligence who need more individually tailored stimulation, and children with dyslexia.

Including children with autism spectrum disorders in normal classrooms where other pupils have been specifically trained to 'reach out' to try to facilitate socialisation and communication with them can be very effective, at least according to formal studies. However, it has to be said that integration without specific measures addressed at helping the individuals with autism spectrum disorders may not necessarily foster any social development.

A small number of children with Asperger syndrome who function intellectually in the normal or low normal range may need the type of schooling which is provided for the 'educationally subnormal' (ESN). It is of the utmost importance that the school system can provide a range of alternatives for people with Asperger syndrome. Some will be functioning well in big groups (provided that the teacher has good knowledge about Asperger syndrome), whereas others will need the 'shelter' of the smaller classroom in which some may have Asperger syndrome and others may have problems associated with other diagnoses. Attending an ESN classroom can be very helpful and, in fact, necessary, in such cases.

Social skills training

Most people with Asperger syndrome, regardless of their level of functioning, need individually tailored training of one kind or another. The word 'training', unfortunately, in some places, has come to mean something negative and has been linked to repressive tendencies in an authoritarian society. Training in Asperger syndrome is usually something very positive, and major gains may be achieved through training, both by the individual and his/her family.

In the whole group of individuals affected by autism spectrum disorders, one working principle is of supreme importance: Nothing (or, in any case, very little) will emerge 'for free', only training will lead to the goal.

It is essential to train people with Asperger syndrome early in life in everyday activities of various kinds. There are often major problems with the things believed by others to be unproblematic: dressing, eating, tending to personal hygiene and caring for the things and order in one's own room. Unless skills in these areas are fostered early, insurmountable problems may emerge in cases with Asperger syndrome. Personal hygiene, in particular, may cause extreme problems, unless a rigorous curriculum is adhered to from early on during development. It may well be one of the most important interventions one can make to implement a curriculum which involves taking a shower (including a hair wash) every day. Such a routine may have to be introduced in the face of there being no absolute need for showering every day. Individuals with Asperger syndrome have difficulty coping with choice situations and it may be that discussing the matter of hair wash every other day introduces just the kind of choice situation with which they are unable to cope.

Training in social skills may be important, but should never be forced in a way which makes it intolerable to the person with Asperger syndrome. The social training should not be seen as a means of 'curing' the basic problem, but rather as a way to facilitate everyday interactions with other people. In school-age children a measure of 'mild force' – or 'authority' – may be called for (and even be perceived by the child as something positive), so long as one keeps an eye on the well-being and negative reactions of the child. Increasing anxiety, restlessness, sleep problems, nightmares or depression might signal that too much pressure is being exercised, and that 'taking the load off' the person with Asperger syndrome, at least for some time, might be indicated. Adolescents and adults should always themselves be consulted regarding their intentions, wishes and needs before any kind of social skills training is begun.

Recent studies have shown that training young children with high-functioning autism spectrum disorders (including Asperger syndrome) in the field of mentalising ability may lead to significant gains in formal mentalising test skills. However, so far, the clinical changes in respect of social interaction have been minor. This is not to say that such training is useless or that it should not be pursued. Rather, the study findings indicate that the 'real life' social interaction problems in autism spectrum disorders are severe and cannot easily be amended through time-restricted interventions – even when these are based on attempts to affect presumed underlying basic deficits. The social/communication deficits in Asperger syndrome are often so severe as to challenge all 'simple' or 'single-faceted' therapies. Even though the 'mind-blindness' encountered in classic cases of autism is usually not present in Asperger syndrome, 'mind vision' is certainly clinically reduced.

Other kinds of training

It is particularly important that social interaction training is not seen as *more* important than other kinds of training or more important than fostering further intellectual growth or the development of special skills. Not so long ago there was a widespread belief that 'social' interventions of various kinds would lead to positive results overall, even in areas that had nothing or little to do with 'sociability'. Experience has shown such theories to be mistaken: social interaction training may lead to some positive changes in respect of social interaction skills – though usually only rather limited changes tend to occur – but in order for positive results to occur in other areas, there is a need for specific training in those areas also. The fact is that training in these areas appears to yield some 'positive side-effects' in the social interaction domains.

Children with special computer skills and interests have recently become 'more acceptable' to their age peers. Many boys and girls without autism spectrum disorders share their computer interest, and so there is sometimes a very good basis for positive long-term interactions. There may be other special interests (e.g. chess, or playing an instrument) and these may well form excellent 'common ground' on which some individuals with Asperger syndrome, eventually, find a 'friend'. It is therefore of the utmost importance to try and find out which special skills he/she is good at. The fostering of these special skills can sometimes be very helpful and pave the way for excellent schooling and vocational training.

Psychotherapies

Psychodynamically oriented psychotherapy not rooted in detailed knowledge about the core problems in Asperger syndrome has no place in treatment. Clinical experience suggests that psychotherapies aimed at trying to implicate childhood traumas as the underlying cause of the symptoms of Asperger syndrome can have devastating consequences. This applies both to the person with Asperger syndrome in therapy, and relatives/significant others who may be indirectly affected by what is at the centre of such therapy. I know a number of adults with Asperger syndrome who have been in 'insight-oriented' psychotherapy for long periods of time, and who, in such therapy, have 'learnt' that the social difficulties and ritualistic behaviours have been caused by problematic relationships with the mother in the first few years of life, by the father's purportedly condescending attitude or by sexual abuse which the patient cannot remember and for which there is no other proof whatsoever. Disruption of family bonds, severe violent acts and social isolation have resulted. In other cases, the person with Asperger syndrome has seen through the clichés offered by the therapist, and, oddly enough, sometimes with mild condescension, decided that the therapy was ineffective and terminated it.

Individual talks

There is often a very positive effect from individual talks with a psychologist, doctor or other people with in-depth knowledge about autism spectrum disorders. In such talks it is important first to listen to the individual's (possibly monologue) story about him/herself, about interests and fears (if indeed a story can at all be shared). Later talks may then be relatively devoid of communication between the patient and the therapist. Gradually the patient may start to home in on some rather concrete problems that he/she would like the therapist's help to sort out: how do you go about making a relationship work, how do you best behave in a group, what is 'normal' behaviour? In such instances, concrete advice is often very helpful. Surprisingly, it may sometimes be good advice to say – after having listened carefully – 'Stop thinking about it!' when the patient goes on and on about a rebuff or a slight, or when he/she worries too much about something he/she did not understand. Obsessive thoughts about death, religion, life's absurdity can darken the life of an individual with Asperger syndrome to the extent that he/she might start making plans 'to put an end to it all'. Telling the patient that you 'don't think that's a good idea at all, much better to persevere and to forget about the bad thoughts' can have strikingly positive effects, leaving the patient feeling much better. On other occasions it is necessary to try to explain exactly why something has happened, something that the patient tells the therapist about and cannot understand at all. Explanations are usually best kept at a concrete level. The level of concreteness required is often astonishing even to somebody who is well acquainted with Asperger syndrome and given the verbosity and level of intelligence of the individual affected.

Teenagers and adults with Asperger syndrome often need individual talks of the kind outlined in the foregoing, particularly during times of distress, depressed mood or social isolation. Also, during times of transition (dwelling, work, loss), regular individual contact is often the best insurance against psychological breakdown (including brief episodes of confusion and psychosis triggered by mild-moderate stress).

It is essential to remember that individuals with Asperger syndrome are not usually 'cold' or 'unfeeling creatures'. To the contrary, their basic affects are sometimes very 'close to the surface'. Their problem is more in their way of dealing with these affects in a cognitive way. Happiness, anger and sadness can all be deeply felt by the individual with Asperger syndrome, but the way he/she shares (or does not share) these affects with other people, is highly atypical. Very often the affects are not shared at all for a long period of time, and then suddenly they erupt in a burst of emotion. In individual talks with a therapist – just as in dyadic relationships in everyday life – people with Asperger syndrome can sometimes get very close to another person, and become dependent on that person's regular contact. The other person may be surprised by this nearness which, in a group setting, would have been regarded as impossible.

Group sessions

Older youngsters and adults with Asperger syndrome may benefit greatly from group meetings with other individuals with similar personality styles and problems. Around the world 'Asperger groups' flourish and are often perceived as extremely helpful (or at least positive) by their members. Occasionally, such a group is best served by having a professional as a leader, but in other instances it is much better to have the doctor, psychologist or education person 'sit in' as a consultant. Some groups work best if there is no professional attending the group meetings. Some Asperger groups meet in order to 'talk', other convene in order to 'do something'.

People with Asperger syndrome (and other high-functioning autism spectrum disorders) seem to be more dependent than other people on spending time with those who share their interests, and have about the same level of intelligence and overall functioning. I have often been surprised by their frank statements that they cannot 'tolerate' those who are not like them, or that they can 'just tolerate' others, but only if they are not expected to converse or interact with them. Clinical experience suggests that Asperger groups may often dissolve if the members of the group are 'too unalike'. One young man attending a 'mixed' group of people with Aspergers syndrome (mixed in terms of intelligence levels and patterns of interest) told me: 'Don't expect me to ever set foot in that group again. The others are so unintelligent, and there is nothing interesting to talk about. They just sit there going on endlessly about their stupid interests. I much prefer my own company.' A year later he was quite pleased with his membership in another group 'where everyone's IQ was above 125'.

In very-high-functioning Asperger groups it may be best for professionals to keep in the background and to participate only at the request of members of the group. However, a certain amount of 'coaxing' and initiative may be required on the part of professionals in the beginning stages in order that the group activities get started in the first place. There is otherwise a considerable risk that nothing will come of the plans to start a group.

Adolescents with high-functioning autism spectrum disorders appear to benefit from group interventions in which the focus is on teaching social skills, including understanding of other people's mental states. However, the gains can be so small from the point of view of the perceptions of others that they may not show in teachers' or parents' evaluations.

On a different note altogether, 'ordinary' group therapy is often contraindicated for individuals with Asperger syndrome. Group therapists need to be aware of this so that they can avoid disastrous consequences of people with Asperger syndrome misunderstanding the interactions, communications and general atmosphere of intensive, out-spoken group therapy sessions. I have met several adults with Asperger syndrome who attended such group therapy sessions and who developed confusional states, broke off all relations with their family and attempted suicide.

Nowadays, many people with Asperger syndrome have found a forum for contact and communication on the Internet. There they can 'chat' – in writing – and interact without having to be literally in personal contact. There are now a number of networks in the field of autism spectrum disorders, and several of these are much appreciated by teenagers and adults with Asperger syndrome. In the future, this way of keeping in contact with other people with autism spectrum disorders will almost definitely develop into an important aspect of quality of life, even for some young children.

Medications

Medication for Asperger syndrome does not exist at the present time, and, in fact, may never become reality. There is currently no unequivocal evidence that any pharmacological treatment successfully and lastingly affects the basic impairments underlying Asperger syndrome. Having said this, it is appropriate to note that the situation is really not different from that in much of psychiatry. Many individuals with so-called personality disorders have more or less chronic, often severe, psychosocial adaptation problems, for which no medication is available. It is also important to remember that while there may be no medication for Asperger syndrome as such, there may be helpful pharmacological treatments available for some of the severe, and common, problems associated with Asperger syndrome, such as depression, obsessive–compulsive phenomena, social phobia, attention deficits and mood swings. It is becoming generally accepted that treatments, be they pharmacological or not, are usually not syndrome-specific. Rather, they should be targeted at particular symptoms, and may be helpful across a range of clinical syndromes.

Neuropsychopharmacological medication in Asperger syndrome should not be prescribed by doctors not well acquainted with the full spectrum of problems associated with that diagnosis.

Serotonin re-uptake inhibitor (SRI) medications

There is a group of pharmacological agents that are often collectively referred to as Serotonin Re-uptake Inhibitors (SRIs). They are also sometimes referred to as Selective Serotonin Re-uptake Inhibitors (SSRIs) to distinguish them from older medications affecting serotonin which tended to be much less specific in their action. However, recent research has shown these drugs not to be as 'specific' as was first believed, and the term SRI is therefore used here, rather than SSRI. The SRIs are also called 'the new antidepressants'.

The most commonly used medications in this group are citalopram, sertraline, fluoxetine, fluvoxamine, and paroxetine. They are effective in the treatment of mild-moderate depression, obsessive–compulsive symptoms and social phobia. These problems are very common in Asperger syndrome, and the SRIs are often quite effective in reducing suffering from these types of problems in individuals with autism spectrum disorders. There is a clinical impression, although not yet upheld by formal studies, that attention deficits may also be positively affected by this class of medication.

There are some side-effects (including drowsiness, mild gastro-intestinal problems, weight gain and aggression) but these are comparatively mild and can usually be reduced to a minimum by starting at very low doses with very small increments every three days or so.

In cases of Asperger syndrome with depressed mood and/or very ritualistic or otherwise obsessive–compulsive phenomena, such medications might be tried, and there is a good chance that clinical benefits will outweigh any possible drawbacks. The patients are often positively surprised that their low mood and severe obsessions could be ameliorated 'so easily'. Even though no well-controlled studies specifically of individuals with Asperger syndrome have been published at the time of going to press, there is now considerable clinical experience suggesting that citalopram, paroxetine, fluoxetine, sertraline and fluvoxamine can all be safely used to affect depression and obsessive–compulsive behaviours in the syndrome. Many clinicians catering to the needs of adolescents and adults with Asperger syndrome have felt that the SRIs may actually be contributing specifically towards the amelioration of the underlying social deficits in high-functioning autism spectrum disorders. This has yet to be corroborated by systematic empirical study, but the clinical impression is so strong that it is now quite common for individuals with Asperger syndrome to be treated with SRIs in an attempt to alleviate the social withdrawal problems.

There is little information about the effects of these drugs on children under age 8 years, and so they should not be used (other than in exceptional cases) in those 7 years or under. I very rarely use these medications in anybody under age 12 years.

It is often a good idea to start with a very low dose (such as 5–10 mg of fluoxetine), increasing every 3 days to a dose at which targeted symptoms are considerably reduced while side-effects (if any) are minor. For depressed mood and social phobia, dosage can often be kept at a very low level (e.g. 10–30 mg fluoxetine daily and corresponding doses for the other agents). For obsessive–compulsive problems, the dose may sometimes have to be increased well above these levels (including to 100 mg fluoxetine or more daily). Treatment needs often to be continued for a year or more. For obsessive–compulsive symptoms, cognitive behaviour therapy should usually be started alongside the medication treatment.

The 'old' antidepressants

The tricyclic antidepressants, now often referred to as 'the old antidepressants' (e.g. imipramine and amitriptyline) are probably more effective than the newer medications for depression. Clomipramine appears to have a particularly marked effect on obsessive–compulsive symptoms.

However, moderately severe and serious side-effects are relatively common and limit the clinical usefulness of this class of medications. Nevertheless, occasionally one of the drugs in this group may be indicated and very helpful, such as in cases with severe depression or very handicapping obsessive–compulsive symptoms.

The new neuroleptics

The so-called 'new neuroleptics' (also referred to as 'atypical neuroleptics'), particularly risperidone and olanzapine, are now commonly used in the treatment of schizophrenic and psychotic symptoms. They exert some of their effects through action on dopaminergic neurons in the brain. Compared to the 'old neuroleptics' (see below), they have fewer severe side-effects, but the very frequent induction of marked weight gain can be an important clinical problem.

These drugs are sometimes very effective in reducing aggression, and can be indicated in Asperger syndrome for this reason. Dosage should be kept to a minimum. Starting doses of 0.5 mg, increasing to no more than 3 mg in teenagers and adults with Asperger syndrome with severe aggressive outbursts are usually well tolerated and sometimes highly effective. For the most part, medication should not be continued for periods longer than a few months – usually so as to accomplish 'the breaking of a vicious circle'.

Drowsiness may be a moderate problem in some individuals, but usually is not severe. Cognition generally does not seem to be negatively affected. Weight gain – perhaps especially with olanzapine medication – is quite common, and, in my experience, becomes a treatment problem, limiting the usefulness of the drugs, in at least every other case.

Clozapine is another 'atypical neuroleptic' which is rarely used in Asperger syndrome, because of its potential to induce blood dyscrasias with life-threatening drops in blood cell counts. In rare instances, it is used, and, when tolerated, can be highly beneficial.

By and large, the new neuroleptics have very few indications in the treatment of Asperger syndrome, but one should keep their anti-aggressive properties in mind and take advantage of these in those, relatively rare, cases in which aggression is the major problem.

The old neuroleptics

The 'old neuroleptics' (also referred to as 'typical neuroleptics'), particularly haloperidol, and thioridazine, are still often used in the treatment of symptoms of schizophrenia, psychosis and tics. They have some documented beneficial effects on stereotypies and social withdrawal in autism, but are rarely used in autism spectrum disorders, because of a relatively high risk of severe neurological side-effects (including cognitive blunting, acute torsion of the neck, chronic inability to sit still and involuntary movements of various body parts, including the tongue and muscles around the mouth). They should be used sparingly, if at all, in Asperger syndrome. Even in cases with acute confusion, which usually respond favourably to treatment with this group of drugs, it is often wise to retain a 'wait-and-see' attitude. Most individuals with Asperger syndrome who develop confusional states recover as soon as psychosocial stressors are removed or decreased. (However, manic episodes, which can occur in Asperger syndrome, do not often respond well to such intervention only.)

When Asperger syndrome is comorbid with severe and debilitating tics, a trial of haloperidol (doses ranging from 0.5–4 mg once a day) may be indicated. In my experience, for this type of symptom, haloperidol is usually well tolerated and effective in reducing both motor (usually) and vocal (sometimes) tics.

Central stimulants

For a long time, the 'general wisdom' was that central stimulants were contraindicated in autism (and, hence, almost by definition, in autism spectrum disorders, including Asperger syndrome). This was based mostly on experience with patients with the combination of autism and severe mental retardation.

New studies have shown that central stimulants can sometimes be very effective in the treatment of severe attention-deficit/hyperactivity symptoms in high-functioning autism spectrum disorders, including Asperger syndrome. One relatively long-term placebo-controlled Swedish study revealed lasting positive effects on such symptoms over a period of 15 months regardless of whether the individual affected had autism spectrum disorders or not. Recommended doses for ADHD are appropriate and should be tried in individuals with Asperger syndrome who have severely handicapping problems in the field of attention, hyperactivity and impulsivity.

Antiepileptic drugs

A small percentage of all those with Asperger syndrome have epilepsy, and some of these will need antiepileptic medication. In my experience, valproic acid and lamotrigine are the two agents that have the least severe side-effects. Carbamazepine, although otherwise often well tolerated, can sometimes lead to more pronounced degrees of ritualism. Drugs from the barbiturate and benzodiazepine groups can lead to hyperactivity, aggression, cognitive blunting and even increase in autistic symptoms. However, in general, the same principles that apply in the treatment of epilepsy in individuals without Asperger syndrome should guide interventions in those affected by the combination of Asperger syndrome and epilepsy.

Lithium

A small group of those with Asperger syndrome are also affected by manic-depressive illness or 'bipolar disorder'. It is sometimes necessary to treat the mood swings with lithium. As with the antiepileptics, principles developed for the treatment of manic-depressive illness generally apply in Asperger syndrome as well. In my experience, the drive for routines and rituals associated with Asperger syndrome can sometimes be very helpful in assuring good compliance with the rather rigorous lithium treatment programme.

Other medications

In autism spectrum disorders there are quite often unexpected reactions to drugs given, such as no response to typical doses, extreme response to small doses or exacerbation of the problems and symptoms targeted by the medication. Clinically, this seems to be true in Asperger syndrome also, meaning that the prescribing physician should keep an open mind regarding matters such as going much under or over the recommended doses, and 'unexpected' or 'impossible descriptions' by patients with Asperger syndrome treated with these medications.

Other interventions

Some young people with Asperger syndrome are greatly helped by intervention programmes prescribed by physiotherapists or occupational therapists. Those who have major problems with clumsiness and awkward gross and fine motor performance or a very unusual type of gait, may need individ-ually tailored motor training programmes. Individuals who are acutely aware of their motor problems and suffer from them should be referred on to a physiotherapist or an occupational therapist, depending on whether gross or fine motor functions are those that are most obviously affected.

Speech therapists with special skills in the field of autism spectrum disorders can sometimes contribute greatly to successful intervention in cases with odd voice characteristics, or whenever talking too loud or too low or just mumbling becomes a major problem. Training in the field of speech/talking may make the affected person much better able to cope with a number of social demands and interactions that previously were felt to be overwhelming.

Concluding remarks

Most individuals with Asperger syndrome need no treatment, at least not in the traditional sense of the word. However, if psychosocial adaptation problems are considerable, a diagnosis should be made and an appropriate examination/work-up performed. A change of attitude and adjustment of the psychosocial environment to the functional impairments typical of each individual with the diagnosis are usually very helpful. Without a proper diagnosis and consequent detailed analysis of the core deficits in each individual with the syndrome it is very difficult for people without in-depth knowledge about the typical cognitive, emotional and behavioural 'style' of autism spectrum disorders to really *understand* how to approach the tack-ling of everyday problems. It is almost impossible to really communicate with somebody who has Asperger syndrome without good insight into the typical cognitive problems associated with the disorder.

A high degree of structure, order and routine in all aspects of life (including, to some extent, leisure time) and a fairly concrete level of communication (even in cases with excellent expressive verbal skills) with few abstractions and little symbolism – these are all important ingredients in everyday work with people who have Asperger syndrome.

The situation at school, or at work, may need to be adjusted/changed in a number of different ways. Assets/strong areas need to be identified and highlighted. Individual talks and group activities – although not based

Table 13.1 Exemplifying list of difficulties, compensational strategies, and self-help skills in a specific child with Asperger syndrome

Difficulties	Compensational strong point	Therapeutic strategy
Selective attention. Shifting focus of attention	Perseverance. Possible visuospatial ability	Introduce simple routines when changing activities: encourage perseverance in other situations than those related to special interests
Comprehend and retain complex information	Memory/TP games, possible visuospatial ability	Write down complex information on cards/ notepads; use Memory-/ TP-kind of games to facilitate rote learning of facts which hold no interest when presented in textbook form
Working memory	Rote memory	A picture or a word for mnemonic support
A tendency for repetitiveness	Unrelenting perseverance, even in situations others perceive as tedious	Progressive introduction of time-consuming and complex activities unrelated to special interests; progressive training in changing activities
Social isolation	Potential for learning to perform independent activities	Organise the time to accommodate *some* social interaction *as well as* independent activities
Verbal communication skills/Conversational skills	Extensive vocabulary; potential visuospatial ability	Write messages, use pictures or concrete objects to illustrate abstract ideas
Compulsive interest in road signs	Strong interest in road signs	Use road signs for teaching the names of colours, shapes, addition, subtraction (e.g. the distance between two points)
Executive functions	Adherence to routines and rituals	Make 'top-10 lists' on items for learning, arrange material from right to left, from top to bottom etc.

Source: Modified after Bristol 1997.

particularly on psychodynamic theory – can be very helpful. Medication plays a relatively minor part in the intervention programme, but may occasionally be of great value for the individual with Asperger syndrome. However, one should keep track of the fact that medication is not indicated for Asperger syndrome itself. It is actually one of the most important cornerstones of 'Asperger syndrome treatment' to steer free of unhelpful medication.

Most important of all is the individualised approach. People with Asperger syndrome have some striking similarities, but above and beyond the problems shared (as a consequence of the syndrome itself), they are first and foremost individuals. In spite of what has been said in the foregoing, stereotyped interventions should not be contemplated. Table 13.1. provides a number of examples of how strengths and difficulties might be identified so that an individualised intervention programme can be tailored to meet the needs of each person with Asperger syndrome. It is always important to remember that there is no such thing as an Asperger person: instead, Asperger syndrome is the diagnosis for a constellation of particular problems that can occur in an individual with any kind of personality, colour, race or persuasion. Therefore, there is no prototype that can be said to be typical of all individuals with the syndrome. Rather, the syndrome is prototypical but the person with the syndrome is an individual! All intervention programmes need to take these basic facts into account.

14

Who can help?

It would have been easy to suggest a referral pattern for autism spectrum disorders, had there existed a service generally expected to cater to the needs of individuals with Asperger syndrome. However, in the absence of such a service it is not a straightforward issue to outline a chain of helpful societal institutions that would know how to provide good diagnostic and intervention guidelines for people with Asperger syndrome. Asperger syndrome knowledge is still patchy and varies widely according to region, training of professionals and whether or not child or adult services are sought. Even when the knowledge is available, organisational and administrative hurdles are abundant in number, making it almost impossible to overcome all the obstacles on the route to help. It is rare for a diagnosis of Asperger syndrome to be made with confidence before the age of 5–6 years. This is not to say that services and pre-schools/day-nurseries need not be well informed about the condition, but rather that education about autism spectrum problems should be directed to schools and school health services (apart from the health services). In the health services, it is paediatrics, developmental medicine, child psychiatry (particularly child neuro-psychiatry), and child neurology that need to be primary targets for educational efforts. However, general practitioners and adult psychiatrists must also be optimally educated. Asperger syndrome is usually a life-long condition and psychiatric problems often ensue. Families, and those affected, may seek help in the general practitioner's office or at the adult psychiatric clinic. Even within services expected to have excellent knowledge in the field – such as in child and adolescent psychiatry – know-how may not be optimal and special educational interventions might be required. In many countries, children and adults with autism (and autism spectrum disorders) are entitled to special help. This is but one of the many reasons why it is important for *all* health services to be aware of the existence of autism spectrum disorders and the basics of diagnosis, work-up and intervention.

Services

A child who may come across as strikingly socially deviant in his/her late toddler or early school years, should alert teachers that well-baby clinics or school health officers need to be contacted. He/she may be thought of as somebody who just will not 'listen', who has strange and fixed ideas or extremely narrow interests, or a very unusual way of communicating with other people. Understanding that such a child is in need of help requires that teachers have enough education about autism spectrum disorders to be able to pick up nuances and extremes of behaviour in children. If a parent raises concern about the child's behaviour at parent–teacher meetings, then the teacher would have to be able to refer that parent – and the child – on to the school doctor, to child psychiatry or developmental medicine. Doctors in these services need to have sufficient diagnostic skills to be able to examine the child, talk with the parent and make a reasonable preliminary assessment as to whether or not the child might be suffering from Asperger syndrome or another high-functioning autism spectrum disorder. If there is a lingering suspicion that cannot be confirmed or disproved by that doctor or his team, then he/she should know where to turn for further evaluation (which could be a more specialised child neuropsychiatrist, a 'specific autism service', a child neurology department or even an interested GP). The important thing is that the child and parents be referred to somebody well acquainted with autism spectrum problems and who has considerable clinical experience in the field.

Quite a number of children and adolescents with Asperger syndrome have developmental problems that will get them referred to developmental paediatricians, or 'habilitation services'. Children who are motor clumsy, or are reported to have 'sensory integration problems' are often worked up by specialists (including physiotherapists and occupational therapists) in such services. Children and adolescents with various kinds of speech and language problems are often assessed in phoniatric or speech pathology clinics. There is a considerable risk that the 'underlying theme' of Asperger syndrome may be missed in such cases, unless there is general knowledge of autism spectrum problems in these kinds of institutions as well as in child and adult psychiatry.

Adults with severe psychiatric problems, extreme relationship problems at work, or who appear to be very deviant either because of a lack of distance or extreme isolation, may give rise to suspicion that they are suffering from Asperger syndrome. Adult psychiatrists, general practitioners and internists, as well as a variety of psychotherapists, should all have sufficient knowledge in the field to be able to make a reasonable decision as to whether the person with the problem is in need of a full diagnostic assessment. Currently, knowledge in the field is so variable and haphazardly distributed that it is impossible to suggest clear guidelines regarding the most appropriate service at which to apply for help.

Over the next several years, health, school and psychological/psychiatric services will almost certainly be better informed about Asperger syndrome and other autism spectrum disorders. It is only when knowledge about these conditions becomes widespread among institutions, out-patient clinics, and the general public, that 'the scene' will change radically. Only then will Asperger syndrome be recognised as a not too uncommon cause of human suffering and misunderstanding. Only then will autism spectrum disorders be correctly diagnosed in the majority of cases, and understood 'in perspective'.

Social networks

The individual with Asperger syndrome, in spite of his/her common tendency for isolation, is more in need of a social network than are most other people. This may seem to contradict the clinical presentation with its dominating feature of egocentricity. However, people with Asperger syndrome are often extremely vulnerable to the ordinary aspects and stresses of life. Only those who know them very well will understand how to furnish an environment that will make life a little easier to cope with. Social networks with sufficient knowledge about the basic features characterising all people with autism spectrum disorders are needed to provide a supportive framework.

It is very typical for people with Asperger syndrome to 'break down' around the time of late adolescence or early adult life. This may spark worries that schizophrenic symptoms are emerging, when, in fact, little other has changed than that the supportive social network has been, or is gradually being, removed. The social network (i.e. the close environment with 'state-of-the-art knowledge' about autism spectrum disorders and the individual with Asperger syndrome) is probably the most important service available. Therefore, the social network needs to be well educated about matters to do with autism, and, hence, enabled to act in support of the person with the syndrome at all times. No (expert) clinical service can outshine the excellence of a well-informed, well-functioning, tight social network, for people with Asperger syndrome.

Support groups

Support groups for people with Asperger syndrome usually work best for adults. In my long experience, it has often been difficult for teenagers to agree on and convene good support groups. However, in adulthood things are often very different; there is both a personally felt need for support that was not there earlier, and the ability to form (and maintain) group activities is much improved.

There are now several excellent adult support groups for individuals with Asperger syndrome. These may function with or without the aid of a professional. It is often wise to have a professional take the initiative when starting the support group, and perhaps be active in the first one, two or three sessions. However, once the group is set in motion, it is usually better for that person to withdraw and to let the support group develop along its own lines, according to the needs and traditions of the individual members.

Concluding remarks

Knowledge about Asperger syndrome and other autism spectrum disorders needs to be disseminated throughout the various communities of the medical profession and clinical psychology. Special expertise must be available in child and adolescent psychiatry (particularly in child neuropsychiatry), adult psychiatry, school health services, and general practice, but also in neuropaediatrics, habilitation services, paediatrics, social services and adult psychiatry. Not until knowledge is well anchored in these institutions will people with Asperger syndrome – be they young children, adolescents or adults – receive an appropriate diagnosis and the kind of help and respect that they are in need of.

15

What about all those famous geniuses?

The 'cases' of a number of famous historical people have recently been 'reopened' with a view to examining whether or not they might have had Asperger syndrome. Among these, Ludwig Wittgenstein is probably currently the best-known 'representative', but many others are 'on the list'. It is always speculative to examine case histories in retrospect, and there can be no 'truth' regarding who 'had' and who 'did not have' Asperger syndrome in cases not clinically examined. Nevertheless, because of the sheer number of publications relating to the possibility that Wittgenstein may have had an autism spectrum disorder, I feel that it is appropriate to elaborate a little bit about him in this book.

Ludwig Wittgenstein

The Austrian philosopher and mathematician Ludwig Wittgenstein is reported to have had a nephew who must have had Asperger syndrome. The writer Thomas Bernhard has described Paul Wittgenstein in such detail (in his book *Wittgenstein's Nephew*) that there can be little doubt about the diagnosis. Paul probably also suffered from bipolar disorder. Bernhard describes Paul and Ludwig as similar in nature.

There are those who claim that Paul Wittgenstein never existed, that he is a fictive person created by Bernhard, and I have not been able to find corroborative evidence of his existence. However, it is clear that many of Wittgenstein's close relatives had extremely odd personalities and that many suffered from affective illnesses. Two of his four brothers definitely committed suicide and another one disappeared from a boat, possibly as a result of suicide. His father was reported to have been very eccentric, attempting to leave home at age 11 years, and then being expelled from school at age 17 after having written an essay denying the immortality of the soul.

In the British daily newspapers in the early 1990s a debate arose addressing the issue of whether or not Ludwig Wittgenstein might have had Asperger syndrome. The Scottish child psychiatrist Sula Wolff has a section in the last chapter of her book 'Loners', in which she describes Wittgenstein as 'schizoid'. Having read this well-informed piece, portions of Ludwig Wittgenstein's 'Secret Diaries', his sister Hermine Wittgenstein's *Family Recollections*, and Gunnar Fredriksson's *Wittgenstein*, I gradually became interested in the possibility that he may indeed have had Asperger syndrome. Talking to friends who knew him slightly (including Iris Murdoch, the novelist and philosopher) and rereading those texts, I now find it likely that Ludwig Wittgenstein had an autism spectrum disorder, and that he fitted almost to perfection the syndrome as outlined by Hans Asperger.

Wittgenstein was born in Vienna in 1889, the youngest of eight children. He died of cancer in Cambridge in 1951, in the home of his doctor, to which he had moved in the terminal stage of his disease. His family was exceptionally rich and very 'cultured'. Johannes Brahms – whose music Wittgenstein liked but felt was 'like a machine' – was a family friend. Many members of the family had strong musical talents. His brother Paul – who lost his right arm in the first world war – was a concert pianist for whom Ravel wrote his famous piano concerto for the left hand.

Ludwig did not speak until well after his fourth birthday. He had continuing spelling difficulties throughout life. Until the age of 14, all his education was provided by private teachers in the family home. He then went to formal school in Linz, where he did well in religion and in English, but not so well in mathematics and physics! Although 'three quarter' Jewish he was raised as a Catholic. He appears to have had great religious concerns in his early years, and was obsessed with feelings of guilt and shame. He was in constant opposition to other people even before adolescence. He later found it very difficult to relate to others, and found it almost intolerable to get along with people from the working classes, because he felt 'wounded' by the crudeness of their company.

He trained at a technical college in Berlin, where he studied engineering, before he went to Manchester as a research student. He went to Trinity college, Cambridge in 1912, to study philosophy (attracted by the writings of Bertrand Russell). There he met one of the very few people, David Pinsent, who was ever really very close to him, and with whom he fell in love (although Pinsent may have been unaware of this).

In 1913 Wittgenstein lived as a recluse in a self-constructed hut on the Norwegian coast. He quickly learned Norwegian. Pinsent died in the first world war. Wittgenstein participated in the war on the Austrian side. There are many stories from this period about his odd behaviours. He appears to have been completely fearless, even during terrible battles, and this gained him several medals. During the war, and later, he was obsessed with the thought of suicide. He was taken prisoner-of-war in Italy, where he wrote much of his *Tractatus Logico-Philosophicus*, which he carried with him in his rucksack. After the war he sent it to Bertrand Russell who saw to it that it was published. He had very close contacts with Russell for many years, but never behaved in a socially acceptable way upon meeting with him.

In 1918, after having given away most of his rather considerable fortune to his family (not to the poor, who might be 'corrupted'), Wittgenstein started to train as a teacher, and then taught elementary schoolchildren in Austria for several years. Parents, children and teachers alike appear to have considered Wittgenstein a big problem. He taught children from poor families, but nevertheless made far-fetched plans for the most talented to go on to expensive higher education, without consulting with the families. The fact that the parents of those children would not be able to afford such education clearly did not deter Wittgenstein. He was very frightening to the children and would sometimes hit them very hard if they did not live up to his expectations. He was probably especially cruel to the less intelligent ones. On one occasion he hit a shy 11-year-old boy who suffered from leukaemia so hard on the head that the boy became unconscious. He panicked, and after having carried the child to the headmaster's room (and awaited the arrival of a doctor), he left the school never to return. A court case was brought after the doctor reported what he had seen, but Wittgenstein was acquitted, most probably because he lied about the extent to which he had 'punished' the boy. Many years later he returned to the area in order to 'apologise', but he only upset the families yet again.

Wittgenstein worked as assistant to a gardener for a while, whereupon he designed and decorated a beautiful, but rather 'stern', building for his sister (who appears as the model on one of Gustav Klimt's best-known paintings) in Vienna (now part of the Bulgarian Embassy).

In 1929, he returned to Cambridge, where he was awarded a PhD and a fellowship at Trinity. In 1939 he was elected to the Cambridge chair of philosophy. In 1947 he resigned and went off to live an isolated life in Ireland. Some of the time there he stayed at the Ross Hotel in Dublin, where the staff grew accustomed to his habit of never having anything other than omelette and coffee. In 1949 he was invited by an old pupil, Norman Malcolm, now professor at Cornell University, to come and stay for a while in Ithaca in the United States. He was already ill, although cancer had not yet been diagnosed. Staying with the Malcolms he insisted on having only rye bread and cheese for his meals. Malcolm once took Wittgenstein along to a seminar. One of the philosophers there, John Nelson, remarked that Wittgenstein looked like a tramp, taken into the warmth on account of Malcolm's generous nature.

During his lifetime, Wittgenstein appears only to have had occasional sexual relations with a few men (and at least one woman), but usually regretted not having 'warm feelings for them'. Much later, he felt remorseful for not having returned the love and warmth extended to him by these people.

Wittgenstein himself wrote that he could often 'not recognise *the humanity* of another human being'; human relations were like Chinese to him, something to be compared to inarticulate gurgling. Pinsent described him as a mixture of oversensitive for his own person but lacking in affection for other people, and Wittgenstein said of himself that he was unable to *give* affection. He was reported to have an endless capacity for finding fault with other people and to be extremely observant of their shortcomings. Russell – and many with him – have attested to his egocentricity, odd dress, naivety, lack of awareness of the presence of other people and of their feelings, but also provided many examples of his 'generosity' as regards money. He would come to other people's homes in the middle of the night, threatening to kill himself, but would then become irritated when they tried to stop him and 'talk him out of it'. Months and years later he would feel remorseful about such behaviours, but in the 'here-and-now' he was unable to 'go outside the narrow boundaries of the self'. Whatever other people might say, even when it was a matter of their personal opinions or feelings, Wittgenstein would interrupt them to say something along the lines of 'No, that's not the point!' or just 'You are wrong.'

Wittgenstein sometimes remarked on his indifference to other people and his inability to perceive of relationships with them in ways that were similar to theirs. He had a concrete sense of humour, but had difficulty with other people's sense of humour. His staring, fixating gaze has been remarked on by several people. It has been suggested that he preferred to be in love with somebody not in love with him, because he could then stay in that relationship 'in splendid isolation'. When other people wanted to be left alone he would come and sit with them, and read to them in an unfeeling monotone, for hours, even when it should have been obvious that they found this very disturbing. He himself would often refuse to have dinner in the company of other people and demanded to be served in his room in private.

Iris Murdoch once (as we were discussing Asperger syndrome) told me that Ludwig Wittgenstein was feared at Cambridge, not least because of his shocking frankness and the lack of any kind of social overtures. In most social settings, you expect some kind of 'social game'; there are usually no 'showdowns' or 'naked clashes' of personalities. She said that he would have none of the social 'stupidities'. He was extremely frightening and she herself – certainly not easily scared – felt terrified just by being near him. She also told me a story – reported to her by a friend of hers who had been present on a specific occasion – about how he could not see the point of telling people why he would be hours late for a meeting. 'Why would I want to do that? I know everything is alright so why would they need to bother?'

Wittgenstein would visit Bertrand Russell and hold endless monologues (literally for hours without allowing anyone into a 'discussion'). He wrote a confession statement about having had sexual relationships with a woman and being three-quarter Jewish, and then read it all aloud in a café – thereby creating a very socially embarrassing situation. He had a number of ritualistic traits. For instance, during the last months of his life, he and his doctor's wife would go to the local pub at 6 o'clock and order two ports. He would poor his into the Aspidistra while she would drink hers! He seemed to find this routine extremely amusing.

In spite of his extremely high intelligence, rigid set of moral rules, and, in spite of being of Jewish descent himself, he seems not to have understood any of the possible consequences of Hitler's rise to power in Germany. He naively applauded men writing disparaging pieces about women.

He came across as pessimistic and often depressed. This would not be surprising considering his family history. However, rather more unexpected may be the observation that he was not usually *really* depressed, and his last words are reported to have been 'Tell them I have had a wonderful life.'

These glimpses from Wittgenstein's life and how others perceived him are sufficient to invoke the typical presentation of Asperger syndrome. It is interesting to reflect upon the very considerable tolerance for 'outsiders' that appears to have been surrounding him for the better part of his life – except during the years when he served as a teacher of primary schoolchildren in Austria. The academic world has long been something of a 'sheltered workshop for the intellectually gifted'. The scene is changing radically in this respect, and it seems unlikely that anybody as 'outside' as Wittgenstein would have gone 'undetected' had he lived today; he would probably now have been diagnosed as having Asperger syndrome.

If Wittgenstein did have Asperger syndrome – what about some other famous people with a drive for social isolation, routines, rituals, and islets of extreme abilities or achievements? There are those who claim that Albert Einstein had an autism spectrum disorder. He had late onset speech, was socially extremely odd and showed a pattern of narrow interests from very early in life. Composers such as Anton Bruckner, Erik Satie and Bela Bartok have been described by biographers and friends/relatives in ways that make it impossible not to consider that they might have had Asperger syndrome. The painter Wassilij Kandinskij is also a 'candidate'. It has even been suggested that the Russian communist leader Lenin may have had Asperger syndrome.

On making a list of famous people who might have had Asperger syndrome, it becomes obvious that their extreme intelligence in one or other area, coupled with rigidity/repetitiveness and social isolation, has led them to the top of their field. From there they may have contributed greatly to good developments, but occasionally to horrendous consequences as well. Most of these well-known people have not come across as 'psychiatric patients' (if there is indeed a 'typical' psychiatric patient). This is important to understand, so that one does not immediately conclude that anybody with the typical features of Asperger syndrome is a 'patient', and one who will have sought psychiatric help.

Concluding remarks

The lives and personalities of a number of famous people – philosophers, composers, scientists and painters – have been described in sufficient detail to allow well-founded speculation that they might have had the typical features of Asperger syndrome. Wittgenstein, in particular, has been described independently by so many different people as having the classic traits. Einstein, Kandinskij, Satie, Bruckner and Bartok are other famous people who possibly had autism spectrum conditions. This is not just an interesting curiosity for experts in the field of autism. The possibility that prominent individuals who have forever put their mark on history in their respective field might have had the condition described by Hans Asperger, is hopeful for all of those whose lives are touched by Asperger syndrome. Maybe one could even speculate that historic progress has quite often been made by people with autism spectrum conditions. The perseverance, drive for perfection, good concrete intelligence, ability to disregard social conventions, and not worry too much about other people's opinions or critiques, could all be seen as advantageous, maybe even a prerequisite for certain forms of new thinking and creativity.

16

Case vignettes

Boy 6 years

Adrian's mother had applied for help at the Child and Adolescent Psychiatric Out-Patient Department because she felt that she had great difficulty attracting his attention. He always seemed to be in a different world and would not tolerate any disturbance when he was active with one of his favourite pastimes. At other times he would just roam about the apartment and seemed never able to calm down. At those times it was really impossible to get him to sit still for even fractions of a minute. Adrian's mother had read about so-called Attention-Deficit/Hyperactivity Disorder (ADHD) in a popular weekly and felt that there were traits of this condition that she recognised in Adrian.

The child psychiatrist noticed at once as she approached the waiting room area that Adrian would not look up from his comic strip magazine even as the nurse announced his name and asked Adrian and his mother to come along to a nearby room. Once in the doctor's office Adrian sat down but appeared to take no interest whatsoever either in the doctor or the mother and continued, sitting in a chair with his legs crossed, to study his magazine intently.

While the child psychiatrist was talking to the mother about Adrian's early development he at first showed no indication he might be listening, but when the mother said that Adrian was extremely good with numbers he suddenly interrupted by yelling out: 'Well, well!' The doctor turned to Adrian with a surprised look only to find that he had already started (resumed) to read his magazine. After a little while he interrupted his reading muttering as though to himself: 'So she thinks you're good with numbers when what you're actually doing is counting; well, well, some things never cease to amaze me but I suppose that's only what you can expect!'

Adrian suddenly got up from his chair and started to walk about the room in an aimless fashion. As he came up to the doctor's desk he put one finger on the top drawing it across the surface and then suddenly withdrawing it as though he might have been burnt, looked at his finger and smelt it. 'Well, well, considerable time has elapsed since this room had the pleasure of the presence of a maid. Ashes to ashes and dust to dust if you please, well, well. You might say that this place is not up for sale but up for dusting. You might equally say that dust is rather similar to dusk, it will soon be dusk and then the dust will be visible no more.' The child psychiatrist considered this for a while and said: 'Yes, I suppose you're right. This room has not been properly cleaned for some time.' Adrian stared straight into her eyes with a disapproving gaze, leaning forward and putting his hands on his hips. 'What do you mean "right"? I would have thought that as a seven-year-old I don't have much of a right, do I?' He then put his finger on the doctor's nose moving it across its ridge and then examining it in a similar fashion as he had just done with the desk less than a minute previously. 'For some time, yea, that's right, for some time, not just the last day or two or three but rather never properly cleaned. So, I suggest you start tidying up at once.' With those words which he pronounced in a sing-song fashion almost like Julie Andrews in the opening scenes of 'Sound of Music' he started to waltz into the room, stopped to do a little pirouette in the middle of the floor before crashing into his chair. A second or two later he was once again deeply absorbed by his magazine. A few minutes later, while the doctor and mother continued their conversation, Adrian abruptly got up and left the room without a word. He stumbled over the threshold but managed to right himself just before falling over. The psychiatrist asked the mother whether it would be best to go and get him back but the mother said he was probably only going to the toilet or into the waiting room area to find another magazine.

Adrian had never showed any interest whatsoever in age peers unless they had piles of magazines in their homes and only if those magazines were among the few he had not already read. He would follow any unfamiliar boy in the area where he lived into his home, into his room, gather all the magazines he could find and disappear out of the house without anybody noticing what had happened. He would also 'bring along' (his own words) magazines from his mother's friend, his father's office, department stores and dustbins. His whole room except where he had his bed was littered with magazines, almost reaching up to the ceiling. From time to time Adrian would 'amuse himself' by building 'brick walls' of all the magazines. He would throw a furious tantrum if anybody entered the room while he was busy with this activity.

Adrian's mother told the child psychiatrist that he had not been able to walk unsupported until the age of 20 months, that he knew the makes of cars and could pronounce them excellently even before his first birthday but that from about the age of 14 or 16 months he had turned almost mute up until the age of almost 3 years. His parents had applied for help at the local GP's, had had his hearing examined and been advised that Adrian probably had normal hearing. Just as they were being referred to a speech therapist, when Adrian was about 3, he suddenly started talking again. In less than a few months his spoken language developed in an unbelievable way so that on his fourth birthday (parts of which were recorded on video tape) he spoke 'almost like an adult, well, at least he sounded like one'. Adrian had a strong tendency to repeat the words that were said to him or that he had picked up by just listening to other people. However, this had become less obvious in the last six months or so even though he had now started repeating some of his own phrases over and over and over again.

Adrian's mother and father had thought of him as very intelligent at least in some areas. For instance, he was extremely observant on details and he appeared to have an exceptionally good memory. His language was very advanced in some aspects but the mother felt that quite often he did not really understand the gist of what other people were talking about. However, the mother's concern was particularly in respect of Adrian's inability to concentrate on things that he himself had not previously shown a particularly strong interest in. When being asked specifically by the child psychiatrist about it, the mother, at heart, was also very worried because of his lack of interest in age peers. A few weeks before coming to see his doctor Adrian's mother had asked him if he did not feel bad about having no friends. His sole response had been: 'No, do you?', whereupon he went back to his magazine.

Adrian had a little brother two years his junior who had started speaking very early and who in so many ways actually seemed to be more mature than Adrian. The mother could not recall anybody in her own or her husband's family who really reminded her of Adrian, at least not as far as his behaviour was concerned. His physical appearance was much like that of his dad, that is if you did not take account of Adrian's squint which was a topic the GP and an ophthalmologist had been discussing for some time, whether it needed to be operated upon or not. Adrian was very slim and it turned out that he was really very fussy about food and he would eat almost nothing except Rice Crispies with skimmed milk and sugar. His head circumference was relatively large but so was that of his dad, according to the mother.

Comments

Adrian shows all the classical symptoms of Asperger Syndrome: lack of interest in other children and a lack of real desire to share and to be with other children, special narrow interests (the collection of magazines), routines and rituals (for instance in connection with the building of 'brick walls'), speech and language peculiarities (late and atypical expressive language development, overly perfect, overly adult language, pragmatic difficulties understanding the meaning and intention of what was being said by other people), non-verbal communication problems, for example as shown while staring at the doctor's nose with hands upon his hips and motor clumsiness (as reflected in his stumbling out of the doctor's office). It is quite possible that Adrian might also have an associated ADHD-type of problem. This kind of 'comorbidity' is very common in Asperger Syndrome.

It is very important that the diagnosis be made in a case like this so that the family and the teachers (and actually Adrian himself) can have the best possible information and gain knowledge about the type and degree of the functional impairments.

Girl 10 years

Brenda stopped speaking when she changed from third to fourth grade in school. She would still whisper to her mother but only at night and only just before going to bed. Both parents, who are teachers, were very interested in fairy tales. They felt that Brenda did right to protest in this way against the 'intolerably hard atmosphere' in her new class. They told her that with so many capitalist families it was not odd at all that Brenda had chosen to be completely silent. 'What could be a more effective way of fighting those vultures?' Brenda's father asked on the family's first visit to the child neuropsychiatry clinic. He smiled in a way which was really rather conde-scending at the intern doctor and said he felt there was a Snow White symbolism in it all. He insisted that Brenda should have immediate 'psychoanalysis', and expressed his opinion that perhaps there was no specialist at the clinic who really had the competence that he himself had in 'evaluating children'. He had been working for two years as a senior high school teacher but for the most part he had been out of work or studying at the university (altogether nine years, mostly astronomy and the philosophy of science, without really obtaining any formal degree). When he left his daughter with the neuropsychologist he said: 'Now finally we'll all get to know whether the frog is a prince or the prince is a grain of wheat.'

The psychiatrist was not able to get a coherent description from the parents regarding Brenda's early development on that first visit. He felt that he had a little better rapport with the mother than with the father, whom he felt had so many different interpretations of the girl's behaviour. He actually was rather relieved when Brenda's father did not show for the following visit. A few days later still the mother came alone and the history that she gave convinced the doctor that Brenda had an autism spectrum disorder.

Brenda had never reacted when her parents or other people tried to attract her attention. The mother had noticed this long before the second birthday, perhaps even before she turned one. She was late walking but spoke relatively early even if the mother felt that there had been difficulties establishing any kind of communication; it was as though Brenda did not really listen. She would talk about her dolls – Barbie and Ken – but would have great difficulty following direct instructions and sometimes actually appear deaf when spoken to.

When Brenda was 6 years of age her parents noticed that she was a collector of marmalade jars. It was by pure coincidence that they discovered that she had lined up more than 30 jars behind the dustbin outside the garage. Her father had thought of this as a sign of Brenda's 'fantastic feeling for outer space' and her wish to move out into the galaxies. Her mother instead had felt a pang of worry, 'like a big black hole in the middle of the universe', but she had not had anybody to talk to even though she had called the 'Women's Alert' and said that she was panicking. The people there had responded by saying that she was most welcome there and had asked if her husband had beat her, raped her or if she had been abused by her boss. When she said that it was all about Brenda, the woman had asked if she felt she needed to speak to a psychiatrist.

Brenda had many ideas. She wanted her mother to tiptoe across the threshold in her bedroom lest she might 'be disturbed'. Her father had heard her say this and wanted the mother never to walk into Brenda's room again because this could make the girl 'disturbed for life'. Father had himself been in 'soul therapy' for two years and had spent more than a year in a camp run by a notorious sect in Nebraska four years previously. He believed he could see right through Brenda's soul and that it was crystal clear and 'elevated'. He would have preferred it if she did not have contact with other people during her preschool years. Brenda insisted that (her) mother put two sugar lumps in every dish being served in the family. At school she was very irritated if the teacher wore glasses because she hated 'broken glass of all kinds'.

The mother told the doctor that Brenda started talking in a reasonably comprehensible way only at about the age of five years. In the beginning she would ask questions only about other people's names and addresses, but she soon turned more interested in the political party they voted for and how many votes were cast for their particular party in a specific community.

Perhaps most incomprehensible of all was Brenda's ability to 'never show her feelings'. She never smiled, never cried or looked puzzled. Dad was very proud of Brenda's 'poker face' and felt that one day she might become a wizard card shark. Mother was more concerned about Brenda's odd gaze behaviours. Brenda would fixate people and stare at them as though she were angry and wanted to show them how little they were worth, only to suddenly look away and appear totally oblivious.

Brenda had problems pouring milk out of the bottle. She insisted on always doing it herself, only to produce a mess on the table, the floor or her own clothes. She would also, after having insisted on dressing herself, come out of her room with a brown shoe on one foot and a blue shoe on the other one.

The mother had read an information leaflet about autism and thought she recognised several of the girl's 'symptoms'. Father, on the other hand, felt that Brenda was only very intelligent, he recognised himself in her and felt that the mother was just unnecessarily concerned. His own mother had been very much like Brenda when he was a child, and he felt that Brenda would turn into something mysteriously wonderful.

Brenda was the couple's only child and neither of them had any experience with small children other than Brenda. When the mother had shown her worries and voiced her concern that Brenda might be 'mad', the father had responded that 'originality is strength, strength is power and power is original'. Mother at first felt that this sounded fine and had agreed not to seek psychiatric help when Brenda was in her preschool years in spite of the fact that staff at her day care centre had recommended such contact several times.

Comments

Brenda had Asperger syndrome. It is possible that her father had the same diagnosis but he had acquired a lot of phrases and interpretations which made it difficult initially to see that he might have the same problems as his daughter. He had great difficulty with reciprocal social interaction with other people, he was fixated on astronomy and he loved neologisms, word games and rhyming. Mother was probably completely well and functioning normally but the number of years with Brenda's father had dulled her reactions to things that in her earlier life she would have perceived as 'abnormal'. Instinctively she had always felt that Brenda was different but her husband had led her to believe that this was not the case.

Boy 12 years

Jason's main interest was glue and paste. He knew everything there was to know about brands, the time they took to dry, and properties and strength concerning various kinds of glue and paste. His parents as well as his teacher had expressed concern that he might develop into a glue-sniffer, but Jason, who had read everything on glue-sniffing, never missed an opportunity to explain to others that 'glue is useful for some purposes, but certainly not for others'.

Jason's teacher had mustered sufficient energy to answer all his queries for years without getting annoyed, but this had become increasingly difficult. Jason never stopped asking questions in class, without raising his hand, and he had also begun to admonish his teacher when she was too slow in replying or when she could not come up with an answer.

For a brief period during third grade Jason had had a 'court' of friends, as his teacher put it, in connection with the school conference she had organised because of Jason's aberrant behaviour. Lately, however, he had kept to himself during breaks, and no one wanted to play with him since he was considered to be 'weird'.

In addition, Jason had thrown a terrible tantrum in fourth grade, without anyone understanding why. He had bitten another child so badly in the ear that he had to be taken to the Children's Clinic to have it stitched. The school nurse had telephoned his mother who, on that occasion, had in fact started to cry.

The school nurse thought that Jason's mother had always seemed over-anxious, and the mother had asked if the boy really seemed all right as early as first grade. However, the school physician who had examined him then had not been able to find anything clearly abnormal. In his health service chart she had written that he suffered from 'a disorder similar to ADHD', with considerable attention deficits and some gross motor clumsiness, although not as severe as to warrant therapy. The mother had said that Jason had learned to walk and speak at a much later age than his brothers and sisters. His teacher in first grade thought that he was adorable, and everyone had seemed at ease with the situation. Even though Jason was an unusual boy he was certainly not in any way 'abnormal'.

Jason had refused to change his desk all through elementary school. His teacher had always managed to move the children from one desk to another in the classroom, but with Jason she had failed entirely. He claimed that the view from his desk was of a special kind and that he would not even consider moving since he then would be sitting at a new angle and would not have the teacher's desk in view. His teacher had found this rather touching and therefore had a hard time abiding by her principle not to let the children make decisions without a reasonable explanation.

Jason spoke so fast that it was often difficult to hear what he was saying. His teacher frequently had to ask him to clarify his answer, and he always repeated his reply without modifying either his tone of voice, content or speed. He was good at geography and history and could name all the major cities worldwide and knew about all the 'important' events which had occurred since 1066 onwards, connecting them with the right year.

A notable feature concerning his historical rote learning was that he could only go from the year of the event to the event itself, but not in the reverse order. Consequently, he was unable to answer the question of what year the battle of Hastings occurred. However, he did know that 1066 was the year the battle of Hastings took place, among various other events. He was useless at mathematics and almost every lesson he got angry and threw his books on the floor and stood by his desk jumping up and down while frowning and emitting a snarling sound.

In fact, both his mother and his teacher agreed that Jason had to 'be sent somewhere in order to get some help'. The only problem was that they could not think of anywhere they believed he would get 'the right kind of help'. Eventually they contacted the school nurse again who suggested he be referred to a children's rehabilitation unit.

Comments

Jason turned out to be suffering from Asperger syndrome. He also met the criteria for DAMP. The children's rehabilitation physician referred him to the Child Neuropsychiatric Team where he underwent a limited examination consisting of psychological and physical testing, including eyesight and hearing tests. In addition, an interview with the mother was carried out as well as a WISC test (see chapter 10), an EEG, a chromosome analysis and a DNA analysis with regard to the FMR-1. The WISC test showed that Jason had a verbal IQ of 122 but a non-verbal IQ of only 88. The EEG demonstrated an increased frequency of slow activity which is often found in DAMP, but no epileptogenic activity. The chromosome analysis and the DNA test both proved to be normal. The mother as well as Jason himself were informed of the diagnoses and both felt relieved to know the reason for Jason's behaviour. He then returned to school and was put in a group of 12 pupils, all of them with Asperger syndrome, DAMP or dyslexia. He began to feel at home and was able to continue in a similar group in secondary school.

Boy 16 years

Dorian was admitted to a correctional institution after having burnt down a day nursery. Though he had first checked that there was no one in the building the night he set fire to the nursery, it was not the first time he had committed arson against a child care institution or public property. During one of the interrogations he declared that public institutions were inhuman and impersonal and added that he did not think one could compare burning down a public institution and committing arson against a private home.

In the correctional institution he was isolated, kept to himself or sat in a corner, usually with his back to the others. Some of the other youths tried to harass him in different ways, but never managed to get any reaction from him, so they soon gave up. He only gave short answers to questions and then in a hoarse, monotonous voice. The consultant thought that he was depressed and suggested therapy with antidepressants. However, Dorian did not want any medication and said he was in a good mood. His face was completely expressionless as he spoke.

Initially he was not even allowed to leave the ward, but he never complained about this. At the beginning of autumn, when several months had passed, he received permission to go for walks with staff from the ward. He then proved a master of all kinds of mushrooms and collected them with great zest and speed. When he got back to his ward he sorted them into bags labelled with the name, taste and distribution of each particular species. He never gave any thought to whether the mushrooms were edible and looked highly puzzled when the warden once made a suggestion to this effect. After a month his room was half filled with bags of mushrooms and he was told to get rid of them. As a result of this request he first suffered terrible fits of rage so that several male members of the staff had to restrain him, and then he burst into tears. 'Take them, then! Just take them! Take all my mushrooms! They'll grow again!' His voice had an extremely monotonous ring to it when uttering this.

Dorian entered puberty late and his voice was only just beginning to break. He was tall with a rather small head, and he looked a bit peculiar even though his facial features were not really abnormal. Ever since the age of three he had been completely obsessed with fire. He had witnessed a fire in the neighbourhood where he lived and, as his father put it, 'never quite got over it'. As soon as the word fire was mentioned or if he caught sight of a matchbox he began to clench his fists and shake all over. He had been a loner from the very beginning and had never socialised with anyone nor had he ever had any friends. His parents had tried to put the matches away and to talk some sense into Dorian, but he only stared blankly at them when they explained to him the dangers of playing with fire. During a period of time they had let Dorian light matches under their supervision, but this had only made matters worse and he became completely obsessed, not only with fire, but also with the smell of burnt sulphur.

Already at the age of 8 he had caused a major fire in a skip and the following year a barn was nearly burnt down after he set fire to the grass some 100 yards away on a day when a strong gale was blowing. His obsession with public institutions – and especially those which had anything to do with children – had not set in until the age of about 14, after a teacher had called him 'childish'.

Comments

The investigation showed that Dorian suffered from Asperger syndrome with a slightly low IQ, in particular the non-verbal level was low, almost reaching the limit for learning disability. The chromosome analysis indicated that this was a case of a disorder called the Klinefelter syndrome, i.e. that he had an extra X chromosome. The chromosomal aberration was the source of his entering puberty late, and probably also of his abnormal behaviour and poor intellectual gifts. Pyromaniac tendencies are rare in Asperger syndrome, but when they occur they require great firmness and absolute prohibitions concerning all kinds of pyrotechnic devices. Prohibitions alone might not prevent a 'pyromaniac development', but a permissive attitude under supervision usually only leads to a stronger obsession.

Dorian will be in need of therapy for many years, first in a 'high security' or 'medium security' unit and then in an appropriate halfway house before the possibility of his living alone without supervision can even be considered. He also needs to be assessed and treated by an endocrinologist, i.e. a physician specialising in hormonal dysfunction.

Man aged 20 years

When Eugene twice within a brief period of time was found at the very top of the tallest bridge in town where he had stood staring out to sea and afterwards said that he would like to know what it felt like to jump, his parents became extremely concerned. His mother had just turned 60 and his father was 68 and had a weak heart: he had suffered two infarctions during the past year.

Eugene's father was convinced that he was of royal descent. He felt akin to Prince Eugene, a nineteenth-century Swedish prince, and considered him to be the best Swedish painter during the previous 200 years.

Eugene was their third child and was, just like his brother and sister, named after royalty. The eldest son, Oscar, who was 34, shared a flat with three other men and around-the-clock staff – he was diagnosed with autism. Eugene's sister, Victoria, was 32 and senior lecturer at an institute of technology. Eugene had always been a model child. His visits to the bridge therefore came as a shock to his parents, who had been sure that Eugene would be successful in life, if he only got an opportunity to develop his artistic talent. His mother promptly made an appointment with a private psychiatrist and Eugene reluctantly went to see him.

However, the psychiatrist did not manage to get Eugene to talk. He only gave a 'yes' or a 'no' in reply to all questions or supplied strictly neutral information on request. The psychiatrist enquired whether Eugene would object to his mother being contacted in order to obtain further information. Eugene had no objections to this as long as they talked exclusively about him and no one else. The reason for the consultation was, after all, as Eugene pointed out, that there was concern for his health, and not for somebody else's.

Eugene's mother saw the psychiatrist a week later. Eugene had, according to her, been very well the past week. The mother said that Eugene's school performance had always been superior except when he had been made to participate in group activities, and when his Swedish teacher in secondary school had demanded that all pupils write a free essay not linked to any concrete subject. As a result of an incident of this kind, Eugene had remained in bed for a week or more, more or less refusing to budge. On one occasion he was relieved of such a task in an unexpected manner. Fifteen minutes after he received the news he was up and out of bed, took a shower and was in excellent spirits. Eugene had also succeeded in being permanently excused from physical education.

His mother, who was a secondary school teacher of English and the History of Swedish Literature, had always considered Eugene to be a 'loner'. He once had a friend with whom he used to play chess, but with whom he otherwise had no contact. He never appeared to be bothered by his lack of intimate friends. However, he was highly valued by his teachers and by elderly people, and no one in his social environment thought much about him being 'abnormal' in any way. Although he was sometimes teased and called 'weirdo' by his classmates, he never paid any attention and it never developed into regular harassment.

His mother also pointed out that Eugene had always been a creature of habit. He would become exceedingly annoyed and sulk for an entire day if some small routine was altered or overlooked. For example, he wanted to be the first to enter a room and became indignant – and perplexed – should anyone else, for example someone who did not know the family, try to 'jump the queue'. Every afternoon around 5 o'clock he would sit in a particular chair in his room to relax. Hence he always became anxious around this time when the family was on vacation abroad and he reminded himself that he did not get his 'chair-rest', of which he considered himself to be in great need. On closer consideration, his mother thought there was a lot in Eugene's older brother's (with autism) behaviour which could also be observed in Eugene. Nevertheless, she was particular about pointing out that Eugene and his brother had never lived together, so any similarities must stem from their gene pool. When discussing this topic his mother became extremely sad.

When Eugene returned a week later the psychiatrist mentioned what his mother had told him. Eugene confirmed everything. He still gave only monosyllabic answers to almost all questions and the psychiatrist began to wonder if Eugene might not after all suffer from depression. However, Eugene denied this vehemently. The doctor then asked why Eugene had visited the bridge. 'Even though I intended to jump, possibly to kill myself, we now are in the middle of trying to solve the mystery of who I am and how could one feel depressed then?!' This was the longest sentence Eugene had uttered in several weeks and the doctor had time to notice that he spoke in a shrill and monotonous tone of voice.

When Eugene returned home his mother asked him what the session had been like. Eugene replied, 'what exactly is it that you want to know?' The mother wanted him to promise never to visit the bridge again and never to try to kill himself. Eugene told her that he could give her such a promise, but this did not mean that he intended to keep it. When his mother said, 'I forbid you to perform another suicide attempt' Eugene nodded and said, 'I will not perform another suicide attempt'. He kept his promise at least during a follow-up period of two years.

Comments

There are strong indications that Eugene suffered from high-functioning autism or Asperger syndrome. This is highly probable since he has a brother with classic autism and Eugene's problems might be found within the same spectrum of disorders. Heredity frequently manifests itself in one member of the family turning out to suffer from Asperger syndrome – often a boy or a man – and another member from full-blown, classic autism.

The psychiatrist obviously had not considered the possibility of his being a case of Asperger syndrome. However, the mother quite soon came into contact with a somewhat younger woman who lived only a few blocks away. From her she received a booklet on Asperger syndrome and realised that Eugene suffered from this condition.

Woman 30 years

Fiona sought psychiatric help owing to fatigue and a feeling of emptiness. She had previously on numerous occasions consulted the local GP due to the same symptoms, but never felt she received any real help. At one time she had been given a prescription for antidepressants. These had provoked such severe side-effects – low pressure and a feeling as if her head was a huge balloon and perhaps also a buzzing sensation in her arms, she didn't quite remember – that she had promised herself never to take any psychophar-macological drugs of any kind whatsoever. On another occasion she had been referred to a psychologist. There she had been offered 'psychotherapy' and she had attended several times, but finally decided that these sessions, which only revolved around the relationship with her sister and her mother, were of no help to her. Of course she believed that most of her troubles were due to the bad relationship she felt she had had with her mother ever since the age of 10, but she drifted further and further into a sense of meaninglessness the more the psychologist kept digging into this particular problem.

During her entire childhood she had had a feeling of being fundamentally different from other people. Even so, she had never voiced the problem in such terms before. A Danish aunt to whom she used to write at Christmas and midsummer had recently sent her a book entitled *Between Autism and Normality* and enclosed a little note on which she had written that the book was about herself and perhaps about Fiona too. Fiona had read it in an almost feverish state and reached the conclusion that her aunt was right. The book was about Asperger's syndrome. Fiona had visited the Library of Medicine and read everything she could find on Asperger's syndrome or 'autistic psychopathy', as she had found it was also called. She preferred the term Asperger's syndrome – or AS as she already had begun to name the disorder. She made a list of the 20 symptoms of the disorder she had found in an English book from 1991. In her own opinion she presented 18 of these symptoms. After the first few days of anxiety and exaltation she had calmed down and had begun to adjust to her new situation. She finally felt 'at home', as she wrote in a brief letter to her aunt. She also mentioned that she had made an appointment with a psychiatrist and that she would write more at length when she had been to see him.

The psychiatrist had read about Asperger's syndrome but had never made the diagnosis himself. He met Fiona three times and then came to the conclusion that she presented a few of the symptoms which might fit the diagnosis but that it was only a matter of 'some traits'. Instead, he believed she suffered from a schizoid personality disorder, possibly obsessive–compulsive personality disorder. Fiona left him with a sense of complete dejection but had already the very same evening decided that the psychiatrist, and not she, was wrong. She wrote a 12 page letter to her aunt summarising her isolated childhood.

Her parents and her sister had always tried to provoke her interest in other children. She took a great interest in languages – at 4 years of age she had tried to learn all words in Swedish as well as in English, French and German. She memorised ready-made phrases, sometimes without understanding their full meaning and without ever using them in social situations. She had had various obsessions – knitting, crocheting, embroidery, Hebrew, Mesopotamia and Greenland – which periodically had absorbed her to such an extent that she had not been able to sleep at night. She remembered how everybody had complained about her when she was younger, that they never understood what she meant, that she always looked 'funny' – or at least not as others expected her to look. She wasn't sure if she was motorically clumsy but maybe she was since she has always detested physical education at school. Her aunt wrote a considerably shorter but nevertheless quite a detailed letter about her problems which in every important aspect corresponded to Fiona's. They decided to jointly seek out a psychiatrist whose name Fiona's aunt had received from a library assistant at work and who, according to a report, had seen quite a lot of autism sufferers.

The two women went abroad and saw the psychiatrist, who confirmed the diagnosis of Asperger's syndrome in both women. The doctor expressed surprise over the fact that they had not contacted the Swedish or Danish experts who had actually written books on autism and Asperger's syndrome. Neither of the women had thought of this possibility and burst into loud laughter when they realised the absurdity of the situation.

Comments

The majority of adult psychiatrists have a limited experience of diagnosing Asperger's syndrome. They are generally more familiar with terms such as schizoid, schizotype and obsessive–compulsive personality disorder. It was not 'wrong' to make a diagnoses of this kind in Fiona's case, since she met the criteria. However, Asperger's syndrome is a more adequate diagnosis since it stems from relatively unaltered conditions with onset during the first childhood years, contrary to diagnoses of personality disorders which should not be made until well into adulthood. Nowadays we also have access to considerably more in-depth literature on Asperger's syndrome than on personality disorders and an ability to communicate with others with the same diagnosis – for example via the Internet – which makes the diagnosis more 'useful'.

It is becoming increasingly common for patients to seek out doctors to ask specifically whether they suffer from Asperger's syndrome. It is therefore of the utmost importance that adult psychiatrists and GPs are well acquainted with the state of the art and with the diagnostics in the field.

Man 52 years

When George had lost 8 kilos, Eva, his wife, thought he had better see a doctor. George had an aversion to all doctors, a feeling he had acquired when at 3 years of age he was put in a children's ward for four days. Hence George refused to consult medical care and it was not until six months later, when he had lost another 10 kilos, that he agreed to see the local GP. The physician suspected he might be suffering from cancer of the colon, but George refused further examination, including X-rays, and the doctor could not force him. Some weeks after the visit to the doctor, George's wife telephoned the GP and told him that there had been a radical change in her husband's behaviour over the last 10 days. He paced up and down in the flat, talked incoherently and screamed at the top of his lungs, flailing his arms simultaneously. Sometimes he sighed repeatedly: 'Oh, Dear God!'

George had stopped eating and now looked emaciated and Eva did not quite know how much fluids he was getting down. The GP contacted the psychiatrist on duty at the psychiatric clinic. The following day George was admitted, against his will, after having been taken there by the social medical officer and a plain-clothes policeman. The certificate read: 'acute schizophreniform psychosis with depressive traits'.

Eva had long since been of the opinion that George's personality was a liability to him, in several areas. He had a tendency to get into disputes with others, especially with his superiors. This belied the fact that basically he appeared to be an uncommonly kind person; that was at least what Eva thought of him. He utterly disdained 'the fawning towards superiors and supervisors'.

The day after being admitted to the psychiatric clinic, George was calm and collected and demanded in a low voice to be discharged since there was nothing psychologically wrong with him. The female senior physician on the ward had had a talk with Eva, who had expressed her concern that her husband had not completed the investigation concerning his weight loss, and persuaded him to stay on for a few days.

The senior physician had several long talks with him. During these George was polite and initially relatively quiet until they reached topics that had to do with leadership, organisation and hierarchy. It became obvious that George's chief interest in life was organisational psychology and he could speak practically without interruption about this favourite topic. He worked as a mechanic in a large company where he performed tasks of a routine nature.

The senior physician initially considered George's intelligence to be high or even very high, at least if one only took into account his way of expressing himself. She listened patiently to him, almost without interrupting, during a whole hour at the second meeting. There was no evidence as to hallucinations or delusions. However, George fixed his gaze straight on the physician's face – nose? – and did not look away for more than a few seconds during the entire session. His mimicry was sparse in spite of his talking in a loud voice and with great intensity. There was a monotonous and somewhat droning quality to his voice.

George was dressed in a three-piece suit and a tie, but had buttoned his jacket the wrong way so that it fitted him badly. The physician made a note in the chart concerning this and that she felt George's outfit to be 'old-fashioned'.

On the third day after his admission George answered to a specific query on the subject that the GP had 'requested an X-ray'. The physician asked why he had refused to undergo such an examination. George replied that he had certainly not refused. The doctor then asked if George now would agree to have a bowel X-ray. George remained pensive for some time and then replied that he probably could not agree to this. When asked why, he did not reply for almost an entire minute while he began stuttering and looking more and more upset. The physician felt concerned that George would again turn 'psychotic' – a piece of information she later entered into the chart. At last he uttered in an almost falsetto voice, 'Don't let them do a bowel rinse on me!' After the talk, the physician informed Eva what George had said.

The following day George asked for a letter of referral for a bowel X-ray. He explained to the doctor that his wife had told him that the GP had not intended to 'rinse out his bowels' but had wanted George to have an enema in preparation for the X-ray.

The examination showed a normal bowel X-ray but also that George suffered from goiter and an over-active thyroid gland. Once medical therapy was initiated he soon began to gain weight and his severe anxiety subsided. He stayed in contact with 'his' psychiatrist, with whom he had become almost obsessed and whom he under no circumstances would part with, despite the fact that he no longer experienced any acute disorder. After a while he was satisfied with an appointment every six months. At these, 'sessions' as he called them, he always talked about his new ideas on organisational psychology.

A year after the acute spell the physician read an article in a scientific journal on Asperger syndrome. She then realised that George suffered from this condition. She informed him of her discovery when they met at the clinic three weeks later. George wished to read the article himself. A week later he wrote a letter to the physician and confirmed that he considered the diagnosis to be correct and that his 'spouse, Eva Eriksson, was of the same opinion' (in George's own words).

Comments

George in all probability, has always suffered from symptoms of Asperger syndrome, even though his disability has been so slight that he has not felt obliged to seek medical attention. In connection with a frightening misunderstanding, concerning the performance of a 'bowel rinse', he experienced a sensation of being paralysed and unable to explain to anyone why he was afraid. He could not imagine that he had misunderstood the GP's recommendation and therefore did not realise that he could ask if that could be the case. To talk about a bowel rinse, even to utter such a word, was unthinkable to him: it was too shameful, revolting and 'dirty'. Only when someone asked him specific, concrete questions about bowel rinsing, which his wife had done as soon as she had been informed by the physician, could the misunderstanding be clarified. It then became obvious that George was not the least bit afraid of the examination, but that he had imagined that his abdomen would be literally rinsed of his bowels by the GP. The somatic symptoms and his severe anxiety subsided after treatment of the hyperthyroidism, but the basic character problems were not at all affected. An IQ test showed that George's intelligence was very uneven with a verbal IQ around 110 and a non-verbal IQ of 74.

Appendix I The ASDI (Asperger Syndrome Diagnostic Interview)

Name of individual rated:

Date of birth:

Age at examination:

Name of informant and relation to individual rated:

Rater:

Date of interview:

This interview is intended for clinicians well acquainted with Asperger syndrome and other disorders in the autism spectrum, even though there is no requirement for 'expertise'. The interview is investigator-based, i.e. the rater is expected to score each item only after determining that he/she has elicited sufficient information for a qualified rating to be made. This means that all the 20 areas listed need to be probed in some detail. Examples of behaviours should be provided by the informant before a rating is assigned. The questions should, if at all possible, be read to the informant as they are written, but may occasionally be slightly reworded in order to assure that the relevant area, of functioning has been adequately covered.

Scores: 0 = does not apply, 1 = applies to some degree or very much

Area 1: severe impairments in reciprocal social interaction (extreme egocentricity)

1. Does he/she exhibit considerable difficulties interacting with peers? 0 1
   If so, in what way?
2. Does he/she exhibit a low degree of concern or a seeming lack of interest in making friends or interacting with peers? 0 1
   If so, please specify:
3. Does he/she have problems appreciating social cues, i.e. does he/she fail to note changes in the social conversation/interaction or to take account of

such changes in his/her ongoing interaction with other people?   0   1
    If so, please describe:

4. Does he/she exhibit socially or emotionally inappropriate behaviours?   0   1
    If so, in what way(s)?

(Two or more scores of 1 = criterion met)

Area 2: all absorbing narrow interest patterns(s)

5. Is there a pattern of interest or a specific interest which takes up so much
of his/her time that time for other activities is clearly restricted?   0   1
    If there is, please comment:

6. Is there a repetitive quality to his/her interest patterns or specific interest? 0   1
    If so, please specify:

7. Are his/her interest patterns based more on rote memory than on true
meaning?   0   1

(One or more scores of 1 = criterion met)

Area 3: imposition of routines, rituals and interests

8. Does he/she try to introduce and impose routines, rituals or interests on
himself/herself in such a way as to produce problems for himself?   0   1
    If so, in what way?

9. Does he/she try to introduce and impose routines, rituals or interests on
himself/herself in such a way as to produce problems for others?   0   1
    If so, please describe:

(One or more scores of 1 = criterion met)

Area 4: speech and. language peculiarities

10. Was his/her language development delayed?   0   1
    If so, please comment:

11. Is his/her language 'superficially perfect' regardless of whether or not
there are comprehension problems or other speech and language
problems?   0   1
    If so, please comment:

12. Is his/her language formal, pedantic or 'overly adult'?   0   1
    If so, please describe:

13. Is there any characteristic about his/her voice (pitch, volume, quality,
intonation, word stress, 'prosody' etc.) which you find peculiar or
unusual?   0   1
    If so, in what way?

14. Are there any comprehension problems (including misinterpretations of literal/implied meanings)?   0   1
    If so, what kind of problems?
    (Three or more scores of 1 = criterion met)

Area 5: non-verbal communication problems

15. Does he/she make limited use of gestures?   0   1
    If so, please comment:
16. Is his/her body language awkward, gauche, clumsy, strange or unusual?   0   1
    If so, please comment:
17. Are his/her facial expressions limited to a rather small repertoire?   0   1
    If so, please describe:
18. Is his/her general expression (including facial) sometimes inappropriate? 0   1
    If so, please describe:
19. Is his/her gaze stiff, strange, peculiar, abnormal or odd?   0   1
    If so, please characterise:
    (One or more scores of 1 = criterion met)

Area 6: motor clumsiness

20. Has he/she been noted to perform poorly on neurodevelopmental examinations either in the past or in connection with the present interview?   0   1
    If so, please comment:
    (Score of 1 = criterion met)

Appendix II The High-Functioning Autism Spectrum Screening Questionnaire (ASSQ)

Name of child .... Date of birth ....

Name of rater .... Date of rating ....

This child stands out as different from other children of his/her age in the following way:

	No	Somewhat	Yes
1. is old-fashioned or precocious	[ ]	[ ]	[ ]
2. is regarded as an 'eccentric professor' by the other children	[ ]	[ ]	[ ]
3. lives somewhat in a world of his/her own with restricted idiosyncratic intellectual interests	[ ]	[ ]	[ ]
4. accumulates facts on certain subjects (good rote memory) but does not really understand the meaning	[ ]	[ ]	[ ]
5. has a literal understanding of ambiguous and metaphoric language	[ ]	[ ]	[ ]
6. has a deviant style of communication with a formal, fussy, 'old-fashioned' or 'robot like' language	[ ]	[ ]	[ ]
7. invents idiosyncratic words and expressions	[ ]	[ ]	[ ]
8. has a different voice or speech	[ ]	[ ]	[ ]
9. expresses sounds involuntarily; clears throat, grunts, smacks, cries or screams			
10. is surprisingly good at some things and surprisingly poor at others	[ ]	[ ]	[ ]
11. uses language freely but fails to make adjustments to fit social contexts or the needs of different listeners	[ ]	[ ]	[ ]
12. lacks empathy	[ ]	[ ]	[ ]
13. makes naïve and embarrassing remarks	[ ]	[ ]	[ ]
14. has a deviant style of gaze	[ ]	[ ]	[ ]

15. wishes to be sociable but fails to make relationships with
    peers   [ ]   [ ]   [ ]
16. can be with other children but only on his/her terms   [ ]   [ ]   [ ]
17. lacks best friend   [ ]   [ ]   [ ]
18. lacks common sense   [ ]   [ ]   [ ]
19. is poor at games: no idea of cooperating in a team, scores
    'own goals'   [ ]   [ ]   [ ]
20. has clumsy, ill-coordinated, ungainly, awkward movements
    or gestures   [ ]   [ ]   [ ]
21. has involuntary face or body movements   [ ]   [ ]   [ ]
22. has difficulties in completing simple daily activities because
    of compulsory repetition of certain actions or thoughts   [ ]   [ ]   [ ]
23. has special routines: insists on no change   [ ]   [ ]   [ ]
24. shows idiosyncratic attachment to objects   [ ]   [ ]   [ ]
25. is bullied by other children   [ ]   [ ]   [ ]
26. has markedly unusual facial expression   [ ]   [ ]   [ ]
27. has markedly unusual posture   [ ]   [ ]   [ ]

Specify reasons other than above:

Appendix III Autistic Spectrum Disorders In Adults Screening Questionnaire (ASDASQ)

ASDASQ ....

Date: ....

Pat. Name: ....

Soc. security number ....

Contact person: ....

Treatment unit: ....

	Yes	No	Don't know
1. Does the patient have any problems regarding contacts with others? (e.g. cannot get or keep friends of the same age, or cannot get reciprocally satisfying contacts with sex partners).	☒	☒	
2. Is the patient odd, eccentric, 'one of a kind'?	☒	☒	
3. Do you find the patient compulsive or rigid, occupied by rituals, routines or rules?	☒	☒	
4. Has the patient trouble with clothing, grooming and personal care? (e.g. conspicuously old-fashioned or ill-fitting clothing.)	☒	☒	
5. Has the patient or has he/she earlier had, special interests, i.e. an intense interest that keeps the patient from engaging in other activities, or an interest that the patient wants to talk about all the time? The subject of the special interest is not important, but the intense engagement or repetitive talking about it is.	☒	☒	
6. Has the patient a bizarre language or strange/unusual voice? Does he/she speak in a very grammatical or old-fashioned way, or use standard phrases or *clichés*, or talk in an unnecessarily loud or low voice? Does he/she talk in a monotonous, or shrill or whining voice?	☒	☒	

	Yes	No	Don't know
7. Has the patient an unusual non-verbal communication, e.g. abnormalities in gaze, gestures or facial expression, unusual posture, stiff gait etc.?	☒	☒	
8. Does the patient seem to have a lack of common sense, or lack the ability to understand and foresee the consequences of his/her doings or sayings? This might cause the patient to repeatedly get into difficult or embarrassing situations, or get others into these situations.	☒	☒	
9. Is the patient uneven in his/her abilities, i.e. very skilful in some areas while lacking elementary knowledge or skills in others?	☒	☒	
10. Has the patient had any contacts with child and adolescent psychiatry?	☒	☒	☒

Further reading

GENERAL

Attwood T (1998) *Asperger's Syndrome: A Guide for Parents and Professionals*. London: Jessica Kingsley Publishers.

Frith U (1989) *Autism: Explaining the Enigma* (p. 204). Oxford: Basil Blackwell.

Frith U (1991) *Autism and Asperger Syndrome* (p. 247). Cambridge: Cambridge University Press.

Gillberg C (1996) *One Child in Every Class: About DAMP/MBD and ADHD* (p. 223). Stockholm: Bokförlaget Cura (in Swedish).

Gillberg C, Coleman M (2000) *The Biology of the Autistic Syndromes*. 3rd edn. London: Mac Keith Press and Cambridge: Cambridge University Press.

Gillberg C, Peeters T (1999) *Autism: Medical and Educational Aspects*. 2nd edn. Antwerp: Whurr Publishers.

Rutter M, Hersov L (1977) *Child Psychiatry, Modern Approaches*. Oxford: Oxford University Press.

Wing L (1996) *The Autism Spectrum: A Guide for Parents and Professionals*. London: Constable and Company Limited.

FOR CHILDREN AND ADOLESCENTS

Gerland G (2000) *Finding Out about Asperger Syndrome: High Functioning Autism and PDD*. London: Jessica Kingsley Publishers.

REFERENCES BY CHAPTER

Chapter 1

Asperger H (1944) Die autistischen Psychopathern im Kindersalter. *Archiv für Psychiatrie und Nervenkrankenheiten* **177**:76–136. In German.

Kanner L (1943) Autistic disturbances of affective contact. *Nervous Child* 2:217–50.

Kanner L (1971) Follow-up study of eleven autistic children originally reported in 1943. *Journal of Autism and Childhood Schizophrenia* 1:119–45.

Klin A (2000) Attributing social meaning to ambiguous visual stimuli in higher-functioning autism and Asperger syndrome: the social attribution task. *Journal of Child Psychology and Psychiatry* 41:831–46.

Ssucharewa GE (1926) Die schizoiden Psychopathien im Kindesalter. *Monatschrift für Psychiatrie und Neurologie* 60:235–61. In German.

Van Krevelen DA (1971) Early infantile autism and autistic psychopathy. *Journal of Autism and Childhood Schizophrenia* 1:82–6.

Wing L (1981) Asperger's syndrome: a clinical account. *Psychological Medicine* 11:115–29.

Wing L (1991) The relationship between Asperger's syndrome and Kanner's autism. In U Frith, *Autism and Asperger syndrome* (pp. 93–121). Cambridge: Cambridge University Press.

Wolff S (1995) *Loners: The Life Path of Unusual Children.* London: Routledge.

Chapter 2

American Psychiatric Association (1994) *Diagnostic and Statistical Manual of Mental Disorders (DSM-IV).* 4th edn. Washington, DC: APA.

Frith U (1991) *Autism and Asperger syndrome* (p. 247). Cambridge: Cambridge University Press.

Gillberg IC, Gillberg C (1989) Asperger syndrome: some epidemiological considerations: a research note. *Journal of Child Psychology and Psychiatry* 30:631–8.

Gillberg C (1991) Clinical and neurobiological aspects of Asperger syndrome in six family studies. In U Frith, *Autism and Asperger Syndrome* (pp. 122–46). Cambridge: Cambridge University Press.

Gillberg C, Hellgren L (1996) Outcome of attention disorders. In S Sandberg, *Hyperactivity Disorders* (pp. 473–99). Cambridge: Cambridge University Press.

Leekam SR, Lopez B, Moore C (2000) Attention and joint attention in pre-school children with autism. *Developmental Psychology* 36:261–73.

Miller JN, Ozonoff S (1997) Did Asperger's cases have Asperger Disorders? A research note. *Journal of Child Psychology and Psychiatry* 38:247–51.

Rapin I et al. (1999) The screening and diagnosis of autistic spectrum disorders. *Journal of Autism and Developmental Disorders* 29:439–84. Review.

Szatmari P, Bartolucci G, Brenner R, Bond S, Rich S (1989) A follow-up study of high-functioning autistic children. *Journal of Autism and Developmental Disorders* 19:213–25.

Szatmari P (1992) A review of the DSM-III-R criteria for autistic disorder. (30 references). *Journal of Autism and Developmental Disorders* **22**:507–23.

Szatmari P (2000) The classification of autism, Asperger's syndrome, and pervasive developmental disorder. *Canadian Journal of Psychiatry* **45**:731–8.

WHO (1990) *International Classification of Diseases and Disorders* (ICD-10). Geneva: Author.

WHO (1992) *The ICD-10 Classification of Mental and Behavioural Disorders: Clinical Descriptions and Guidelines.* Geneva: WHO.

WHO (1993) *The ICD-10 Classification of Mental and Behavioural Disorders: Diagnostic Criteria for Research.* Geneva: WHO.

Wing L (1981) Asperger's syndrome: a clinical account. *Psychological Medicine* **11**:115–29.

Chapter 3

Chakrabarti S, Fombonne E (2001) Pervasive developmental disorders in preschool children. *Journal of the American Association* **27**; 285, 3093–9.

Ehlers S, Gillberg C (1993) The epidemiology of Asperger syndrome: a total population study. *Journal of Child Psychology and Psychiatry* **34**:1327–50.

Gillberg C (1995) *Clinical Child Neuropsychiatry* (p. 366). Cambridge and New York: Cambridge University Press.

Gillberg C, Wing L (1999) Autism: not an extremely rare disorder. *Acta Psychiatrica Scandinavica* **99**:399–406. Review.

Gillberg IC, Gillberg C (1989) Asperger syndrome. Some epidemiological considerations: a research note. *Journal of Child Psychology and Psychiatry* **30**: 631–8.

Gillberg C (1991) Clinical and neurobiological aspects of Asperger syndrome in six family studies. In U Frith, *Autism and Asperger Syndrome* (pp. 122–46). Cambridge: Cambridge University Press.

Kadesjö B, Gillberg C, Hagberg B (1999) Brief report: autism and Asperger syndrome in seven-year-old children: a total population study. *Journal of Autism and Developmental Disorders* **29**:327–31.

Landgren M, Kjellman B, Gillberg C (1996) ADHD, DAMP and other neurodevelopmental/neuropsychiatric disorders in six-year-old children: epidemiology and comorbidity. *Developmental Medicine and Child Neurology* **38**:891–906.

Lesinskiene S, Puras D (2001) Prevalance of Asperger syndrome among children of Vilnius. *International Journal of Circumpolar Health* **60**:(suppl.), 13.

Nylander L, Gillberg C (2001) Screening for autism spectrum disorders in adult psychiatric outpatients: A preliminary report. *Acta Psychiatrica Scandinavica* **103**:428–34.

Wing L (1996) *The Autistic Spectrum.* London: Constable.

Chapter 4

Asperger H (1979) Problems of infantile autism. *Communication* **13**:45–52.

Gerland G (1997) *A Real Person: Life on the Outside.* London: Souvenir Press.

Gillberg C (1990) Hans Asperger: an unreachable individual. *Läkartidningen* **87**:2973. In Swedish, summary in English.

Grandin T (1983) Coping strategies (letter). *Journal of Autism and Developmental Disorders* **13**:217–22.

Hewett E, Newson E, Newson J (1970) *The Family and the Handicapped Child.* London: Allen & Unwin.

Newson E (1983) Pathological demand-avoider syndrome. *Communication* **17**:3–8.

Newson J, Newson E (1970) The handicapped child: what is an autistic child? *Nursing Times* **75**:(suppl.), 4–5.

Sacks O (1995) *An Anthropologist on Mars: Seven Paradoxical Tales.* London: Picador Books.

Wing L (1989) The diagnosis of autism. In Gillberg C. *Diagnosis and Treatment of Autism.* New York, Plenum Press, pp. 5–22.

Chapter 5

Tantam D (1988) Asperger's syndrome. *Journal of Child Psychology and Psychiatry* **29**:245–55.

Wing L (1989) Autistic adults. In C Gillberg, *Diagnosis and Treatment of Autism* (pp. 419–32). New York: Plenum Press.

Wolff S, Chick J (1980) Schizoid personality in childhood: a controlled follow-up study. *Psychological Medicine* **10**:85–100.

Schäfer S (1997) *Sterne, Äpfel und rundes Glas: mein Leben mit Autismus.* Stuttgart: Verlag Freies Geistesleben.

Szatmari P, Bryson SE, Streiner DL et al. (2000) Two-year outcome of pre-school children with autism or Asperger's syndrome. *American Journal of Psychiatry* **157**:1980–7.

Chapter 6

Kadesjö B, Gillberg C (1999) Developmental co-ordination disorder in Swedish 7-year-old children. *Journal of the American Academy of Child and Adolescent Psychiatry* **38**:820–8.

Kadesjö B, Gillberg C (2000) Tourette's disorder: epidemiology and comorbidity in primary school children. *Journal of the American Academy of Child and Adolescent Psychiatry* **39**:548–55.

Tatam D (1991) Asperger syndrome in adulthood. In U Frith (ed.), *Autism and Asperger syndrome* (pp. 147–83). Cambridge: Cambridge University Press.

Wentz E, Gillberg C, Gillberg CI, Råstam M (2001) Ten-year follow-up of adolescent-onset anorexia nervosa: psychiatric disorders and overall functioning scales. *Journal of Child Psychology and Psychiatry*. In press.

Wing L (1981) Asperger's syndrome: a clinical account. *Psychological Medicine* 11:115–29.

Wing L, Shah A (2000) Catatonia in autistic spectrum disorders.
British Journal of Psychiatry 176:357–62.

Chapter 7

Gillberg C (1989) Asperger syndrome in 23 Swedish children. *Developmental Medicine and Child Neurology* 31:520–31.

Gillberg C, Billstedt E (2000) Autism and Asperger syndrome: coexistence with other clinical disorders. *Acta Psychiatrica Scandinavica* 102:321–30.

Chapter 8

Gillberg C (1991) Clinical and neurobiological aspects of Asperger syndrome in six family studies. In U Frith (ed.), *Autism and Asperger Syndrome*. Cambridge: Cambridge University Press.

Hermelin B, O'Connor N (1970) *Psychological Experiments with Autistic Children*. Oxford: Pergamon Press.

Sacks O (1994) A neurologist's notebook: an anthropologist on Mars. *The New Yorker* 3:106–25.

Chapter 9

Beversdorf DO et al. (2000) Increased discrimination of 'false memories' in autism spectrum disorder. *Proceedings of the National Academy of Sciences of the United States of America* 18:97: 8734–7.

Baron-Cohen S, Ring HA, Wheelwright S et al. (1999) Social intelligence in the normal and autistic brain: an fMRI study. *European Journal of Neuroscience* 11:1891–8.

Critchley HD, Daly EM, Bullmore ET et al. (2000) The functional neuroanatomy of social behaviour: changes in cerebral blood flow when people with autistic disorder process facial expressions. *Brain*. Nov.: 123 (pt. 11): 2203–12.

Gillberg C (1999) Neurodevelopmental processes and psychological functioning in autism. *Developmental Psychopathology* 11:567–87. Review.

Gillberg C, Coleman M (2000) *The Biology of the Autistic Syndromes*. 3rd edn. London:

Mac Keith Press and Cambridge: Cambridge University Press.

Happé F, Ehlers S, Fletcher P et al. (1996) 'Theory of mind' in the brain: evidence from a PET scan study of Asperger syndrome. *NeuroReport* **8**(1): 197–201.

Haznedar MM, Buchsbaum MS, Wei TC et al. (2000) Limbic circuitry in patients with autism spectrum disorders studied with positron emission tomography and magnetic resonance imaging. *American Journal of Psychiatry* **157**:1994–2001.

Ring HA, Baron-Cohen S, Wheelwright S et al. (1999) Cerebral correlates of preserved cognitive skills in autism: a functional MRI study of embedded figures task performance. *Brain* **122**:1305–15.

Schultz RT, Gauthier I, Klin A, et al. (2000) Abnormal ventral temporal cortical activity during face discrimination among individuals with autism and Asperger syndrome. *Archives of General Psychiatry* **57**(4): 331–40.

Taylor DC, Neville BG, Cross JH (1999) Autistic spectrum disorders in childhood epilepsy surgery candidates. *European Child Adolescent Psychiatry*. Sept. **8**(3): 189–92.

Chapter 10

Baron-Cohen S (1995) *Mind Blindness: An Essay on Autism and Theory of Mind.* Cambridge, MA: MIT Press.

Baron-Cohen S, Leslie AM, Frith U (1986) Mechanical, behavioural and intentional understanding of picture stories in autistic children. *British Journal of Developmental Psychology* 113–25.

Dewey M (1991) *Living with Asperger's syndrome: Autism and Asperger syndrome* (pp. 184–206). U Frith ed. Cambridge: Cambridge University Press.

Ehlers S, Gillberg C, Wing L (1998) A screening questionnaire for Asperger syndrome and other high-functioning autism spectrum disorders in school age children. *Journal of Autism and Developmental Disorders* **29**:129–41.

Ehlers S, Nydén A, Gillberg C et al. (1997) Asperger syndrome, autism and attention disorders: a comparative study of the cognitive profile of 120 children. *Journal of Child Psychology and Psychiatry* **38**:207–17.

Frith U (1989) *Autism: Explaining the Enigma.* Oxford: Basil Blackwell.

Happé FGE (1994a) Wechsler IQ profile and theory of mind in autism: a research note. *Journal of Child Psychology and Psychiatry* **35**:1461–71.

Happé FGE (1994b) An advanced test of theory of mind: understanding of story characters' thoughts and feelings by able autistic, mentally handicapped, and normal children and adults. *Journal of Autism and Developmental Disorders* **24**:129–54.

Happé FGE (1994c) Current psychological theories of autism: the 'Theory of Mind' accountant and rival theories. *Journal of Child Psychology and Psychiatry* **35**:215–29.

Hughes CM, Leboyer M, Bouvard M (1997) Executive function in parents and children with autism. *Psychosocial Medicine* **27**(1): 209–20.

Klin A (1997) Asperger syndrome and non-verbal learning disabilities: imaging, brain diagnostic and medical findings. LDA International Conference. Chicago, IL. 19–22 February, 1997.

Nydén A, Gillberg C, Hjelmquist E, Heiman M (1999) Executive function/attention in boys with Asperger syndrome, attention disorders and reading/writing disorder. *Autism* **3**:213–28.

Pennington BF, Ozonoff S (1996) Executive functions and developmental psychopathology. *Journal of Child Psychology and Psychiatry* **37**:51–87.

Rapin I (ed.) (1996) *Preschool Children With Inadequate Communication: Development Language Disorder, Autism, Mental Deficiency. Clinics in Developmental Medicine No. 139.* London: Mac Keith Press, with Cambridge University Press.

Temple CM (1997) Cognitive neuropsychology and its application to children. *Journal of Child Psychology and Psychiatry* **38**:27–52.

Chapter 11

Ehlers S, Gillberg C (1993) The epidemiology of Asperger syndrome. A total population study. *Journal of Child Psychology and Psychiatry* **34**:1327–50.

Gillberg C, Coleman M (2000) *The Biology of the Autistic Syndromes,* 3rd revd edn. Clinics in Developmental Medicine No. 153/4. London, New York: Mac Keith Press and Cambridge: Cambridge University Press.

Gilberg C, Gillberg IC, Råstam M, Wentz E (2001) The Asperger Syndrome Diagnostic Interview (ASDI): a new structured interview for use in clinical practice. *Autism* **5**:57–66.

Nylander L, Gillberg C (2001) Screening for autism spectrum disorders in adult psychiatric out-patients: a preliminary report. *Acta Psychiatrica Scandinavica* **103**:428–34.

Prior M, Eisenmajer R, Leekam S et al. (1998) Are there subgroups within the autistic spectrum? A cluster analysis of a group of children with autistic spectrum disorders. *Journal of Child Psychology and Psychiatry* **39**:893–902.

Filipek PA, Accardo PJ, Baranek GT et al. (1999) The screening and diagnosis of autistic spectrum disorders. *Journal of Autism and Developmental Disorders* **29**:439–84. Review.

Lord C, Rutter M, Le Couteur A (1994) Autism Diagnostic Interview – Revised: A revised version of a diagnostic interview for caregivers of individuals with possible pervasive developmental disorders. *Journal of Autism and Developmental Disorders* **24**:659–85.

Wing L, Leekham L, Libby S et al. (2002) The Diagnostic Interview for Social and Communication Disorders: background, inter-rater reliability and clinical use. *Journal of Child Psychology and Psychiatry* **43**.

Chapter 12

Bristol M (1997) Interventions in Asperger Syndrome. In Paper given at the Learning Disabilities Association International Conference. Chicago (19–22 February) *Journal of Autism and Developmental Disorders*. Special Issue on Treatment 2000.

Gillberg C, Ehlers S (1998) High-functioning people with autism and Asperger syndrome: a literature review. In E Schopler, G Mesibov, Kunce *Asperger Syndrome or High Functioning Autism?* Special Issue of Journal of Autism and Developmental Disorders (pp. 79–106). New York: Plenum Press.

Nordin V, Gillberg C (1998) The long-term course of autistic disorders: update on follow-up studies. (Review) *Acta Psychiatrica Scandinavica* **97**:99–108.

Scragg P, Shah A (1994) Prevalence of Asperger's syndrome in a secure hospital. *British Journal of Psychiatry* **165**:679–82.

Szatmari P, Bryson SE, Streiner DL et al. (2000) Two-year outcome of preschool children with autism or Asperger's syndrome. *American Journal of Psychiatry* **157**:1980–7.

Tantam D (1993) The developmental psychopathology of emotional disorders. (Review) (14 references). *Journal of the Royal Society of Medicine* **86**:336–40.

Tantam D, Holmes D, Cordess C (1993) Non-verbal expression in autism of Asperger type. *Journal of Autism and Developmental Disorders* **23**:111–33.

Chapter 13

Gillberg C, Nordin V, Ehlers S (1996) Early detection of autism: diagnostic instruments for clinicians. *European Child and Adolescent Psychiatry* **5**:67–74.

Mesibov GB (1995) Commentary: facilitated communication: a warning for pediatric psychologists. *Journal of Pediatric Psychology* **20**:127–30.

Chapter 14

Hellström A (1995) *Now it's Our Turn: How to Support Children with MBD/DAMP*. Stockholm: RBU (The National Society for Disabled Children and Adolescents)/ Liber Utbildning. In Swedish.

Chapter 15

Bernhard T (1982) *Wittgenstein's Neffe: Eine Freundschaft*. Frankfurt-am-Main: Suhrkamp Verlag.

Fredriksson G (1993) *Wittgenstein*. Stockholm: Albert Bonniers Förlag. In Swedish.

Murdoch I (1989) *The Message to the Planet*. London: Chatto & Windus.

Wolff S (1995) *Loners: The Life Path of Unusual Children*. London: Routledge.

Index